MW01256992

i

Victory

Over

Depression

With and Without Medicines

Bergina Isbell, MD

To the loves of my life,

Amir Sr, J'Pia, and Amir Jr

ISBN: 978-0-9987553-0-4

Acknowledgments

Though I love to read, I did not have a full appreciation for how much work actually goes into the creation and development of a book. I would not have been able to complete this book without the help of a great team. Although an entire book itself could be written to thank the many people that contributed to bringing this book out of my office and into your hands, I will be as brief as possible.

First, Father, I thank you for your wisdom, guidance, and strength. You are my best encourager!

To my husband, Dr. Amir, thank you for everything you have done to get this book to a publishable format. From sharing your knowledge as a medical researcher, to providing a safe place to write and air my ideas (and complaints), you sacrificed much time and sleep. I thank you so very much.

Thank you to every patient that entrusted your stories to me and helped provide the basis for the contents of this book. As I have shared with you before, it has been my honor that you invited me to travel with you on your journey.

Pastor Yusef Fletcher and Coach Mia Redrick, I thank you both for planting the idea of writing down what I share with my patients every day. Dr. Kahlil Johnson, thank you for your medical review and reminder of the basic writing techniques that we all learned in school so many years ago. Carol Trupe, I greatly appreciate your teaching of Cognitive Behavior Therapy techniques as well as your faithful review of my attempts to put it into writing.

Donna Koczaja and Angela "Violet" Keys, you both provided a wealth of information about herbals and essential oils. Thank you for willingness to share your expertise.

To my family, friends, colleagues, and partners, thank you for your generous support.

Finally, to the reader, thank you. You too have contributed to "the reason behind the reason" for the writing of this book. A portion of the proceeds of all of my books are given back to non-profit organizations providing help to others with mental health concerns.

Table of Contents

Introduction

When you are dealing with any disease, whether it is high blood pressure, diabetes, or depression, you first have to know that you actually have the disease. As philosopher Francis Bacon said, "Knowledge itself is power." The purpose of this book is to help inform you about depression and to provide an understanding about the options to treat it. My sincerest hope is that you will move from knowledge to understanding, and then from understanding to wisdom.

Many of my patients come to me for the knowledge that I have, in hopes that I have information that can help them better understand why they feel so badly. While my knowledge base helps me determine fairly accurately which disorder they may have and what treatment option to pursue, this is only part of the story. The difference between the science of medicine and the art of medicine, in my mind, is wisdom. Wisdom helps with determining things that are not evident in a treatment flow diagram. Things like timing, patience, and empowerment are not as easily taught.

As we journey towards a better understanding of depression and options you have for treatment, I share my knowledge with you, but more importantly, I attempt to share wisdom as well.

While I acknowledge that some of my wisdom comes from a Christian worldview, I want to be very clear that many illnesses, including depression, know no religious, racial, gender, or economic boundaries.

In fact, the World Health Organization estimates 350 million people suffer from depression globally. Depression is the leading cause of disability worldwide (WHO, 2016). I am one of those who have had a diagnosis of Major Depressive Disorder, or clinical depression. This is a diagnosis associated with an enormous burden of loss of activity and function, or death. Sadly, many of these millions have not had the experience I had of having it diagnosed and treated until it was entirely resolved (medically referred to as complete remission).

We have all felt saddened by a loss, or felt a depressed mood related to a disappointment. A wise man, Dr. Kowatch wrote, "Not all mood swings are bipolar disorder." Likewise, all sad moods are not depression. Some people have labeled the normal spectrum of human emotions we have been gifted with as illness. But a medical diagnosis of Major Depressive Disorder is something different.

My training helped me to acknowledge that I was experiencing a clinical depression. Once I did recognize the various symptoms, I had to decide what I was going to do about it. I sought treatment.

I began to see a Psychotherapist. I was honored to be a part of a Residency program at the Mayo Clinic that actively sought to prevent medical providers, who treat people with mental illnesses, from falling prey to depression and other mental illnesses.

Opportunities have been in place at least since Dr. Sigmund Freud pioneered the field of Psychiatry in the late 1890s for both training and established Psychiatrists to help keep them from becoming overwhelmed by the work they do. In the 1960s, Psychiatrists had to attend mandatory psychotherapy (commonly referred to as "talk therapy"). You still see this in doctors training in the more traditional fields of psychotherapy (i.e. Psycho-dynamic Psychotherapy, or Psychoanalytic Psychotherapy).

Nowadays, even if mandatory therapy is not a requirement, resident physicians (Psychiatrists in-training) are required to have at least one psychotherapy supervisor. In my training program we had two - one for review of patients' pharmacological treatment, and another for review of patient's psychotherapy treatment. In addition to that, we met weekly in a group to discuss our psychotherapy cases. We were given multiple opportunities to process difficult cases. For example, we discussed personal and case related difficult feelings, what we call counter-transference, or feelings that you might be picking up from a patient.

Although I started with psychotherapy, when the depression became more severe for me, my Psychiatrist, who happened to be a Christian, recommended medication. Some cultures and religions do not believe in medications for depression, so this is of importance for many who may struggle with a decision to seek care. In both my culture and my faith community, acknowledging depression and seeking treatment can be difficult. Additionally, several of my medical colleagues have found it difficult to seek care for certain disorders due to the stigma associated with them.

One of my favorite places has always been the library, and I would often sit in our trainee library surrounded by meticulously labeled and catalogued texts. I was both grateful and a bit surprised by how many books, memoirs, and audio material there was on clinicians who dealt with mental illness themselves. While some clinicians who have dealt with mental illness have decided not to treat patients clinically, there are many, including myself who have. I think it helps my patients to know that I have been where they are, and that recovery is possible. The advantage of being a resident in psychiatry is that it made it easier for me to seek treatment. It will be my privilege to help you do the same.

CHAPTER 1

Recognize That You Are Dealing With Depression

"Why art thou downcast, Oh my soul? Why art thou disquieted within me...?"

-King David

Looking back, I can tell from pictures the year my depressive symptoms began. When flipping through family albums, I see a little girl with ponytails and chubby cheeks, smiling at the camera. Sometimes I have no front teeth and at other times, no bangs or curls in my hair. But that same smile, the same light in my eyes is there. At least until my fifth- grade year. Sometime that year it happened. I can tell because the smile dimmed, was almost forced. One could think it was simply a little girl being self-conscious about her now slightly crooked teeth. But to arrive at that opinion you would have to have missed her eyes. I can see it. The sparkle was gone. The Sadness was present, hidden, but there.

When I was a Resident Physician in Psychiatry at the Mayo Clinic, one of my professors described depression as a "cancer of the soul." Like cancer, depression starts insidiously. It begins slowly, yet causes pain and suffering from the very start. You find yourself more tired than normal; your energy sapped for no reason. You have little appetite, no longer finding joy and satisfaction in either the food you eat or the things you used to do. You isolate from others, preferring to be alone because conversations have become so meaningless, and you cannot keep up with what people are saying anyway.

Did you used to have good times? Remembering things takes effort. Your focus is off. You are off your game. You think, maybe you just need more sleep, but you have been sleeping more and more. Or perhaps, your sleep varies. Sometimes, you feel that all you want to do is sleep. Other times, you toss and turn at night watching the clock go from 2 o'clock to 3 o'clock to 4 o'clock. If you finally fall asleep, leaving the comfort of your bed becomes drudgery. The bright light streaming in on a new day is an intrusion. "What is going on?!?," you ask.

Now, at this point you are maybe getting a little angry, a little irritable. Others begin to see it and comment on it. Your responses are terse, and you are short with people. They steer clear of you, you isolate even more, and the cycle continues. Left alone, the sickness lingers. For some, the illness can kill.

Some patients can tell me exactly when their depression began. For example, they can pinpoint it to a financial crisis, or while going through a divorce. They know when they went from being happy and fulfilled, to looking at life through fecal colored glasses. Others can share time after time of struggle across a broad range of suffering. People's struggles have stemmed from being a child living in poverty, being bullied as a teen, or a stressful life working in a job that pays too little but asks for everything. For many, the depression slipped in unannounced and initially unnoticed.

I know there are many that continue to struggle quietly with depression due to stigma. Depression can be a time limited illness for some, and the natural history of the disease is such that it can peak, fade, and completely regress with little to no intervention. So, for many, they cope with their depression on their own. Others, begin the process of working with a mental health professional, but for many reasons, do not continue treatment until they improve. Often, the precipitant for the depression is the culprit, the reason for leaving treatment. For example, job stress precipitates the depression, but patients cannot find time away from the job to come to appointments. Many begin following the treatment plan that has been outlined for them, but pill burden (taking a large number of medications), side effects, or interactions with their other medicines cause them to stop treatment. They may or may not share this with their doctor or treatment provider. Some start getting better, but then notice that they only return to a shadow of their former selves or former level of functioning and are dissatisfied with their current state of living.

If you are dealing with depression, you are certainly not alone. As discussed in the Introduction, 350 million people worldwide suffer from depression, according to the World Health Organization. Many people have struggled with this illness in various forms for centuries. Two very prolific stories involving depression are reflected in the accounts of King David and Job (pronounced "Jobe"). In both stories, they dealt with a depressed state, and likely, clinical depression. The story of King David is exemplary at providing an example of how to overcome depression, while Job's is a perfect example of what depression looks like.

But, before we get to Job's depression, let's deal with the initial symptom with which he presented. He first experienced one of many popular masqueraders of depression - grief. Job literally lost everything he had in one day, from all of several thousands of his cattle, sheep, and other livestock and business, to the death of his children. He described his emotions quite

10

eloquently in regard to his grief. In the book of Job, he said "all that my grief are actually weighed and laid in the balances together with my calamity." He grieved the loss of his children as well as the terrible situation in which he found himself.

While there is no particular cut off or timeline for when a person who is sad or down as a result of a loss of family member is expected to grieve, often I have been referred patients who are dealing only with grief, or Uncomplicated Bereavement, and not depression. It is to be expected that a person may feel sad and lonely after the death of a loved one. They may experience appetite or sleep changes as well. Some patients have even shared with me they hear their name being called by their beloved deceased spouse. This can occur in Bereavement, the medical name for grief, depending on the circumstances of the death.

Now, if this is all that Job experienced, I would have diagnosed him with Uncomplicated Bereavement. But, what Job experienced does not stop there. He shared several more symptoms that are more so in line with depression than grief alone. He described himself as "a despairing man" and his spirit as "broken." He experienced appetite changes where things were "tasteless" which he likened to eating the white of the egg without salt and his "groaning" at the sight of food. He has experienced some form of weight loss, and likely energy loss, and described his body as "decaying" and "shriveled." He was tearful saying that his face was "flush with weeping" and lamented that his "cries pour out like water." Job certainly experienced a loss of interest in spending time with his friends. When they came to comfort him, they all sat for seven days and seven nights in silence because of his great pain. He talked of the intense emotional pain he experienced. He experienced insomnia and "longs for sleep." He said, "I would have lain down and been quiet. I would have slept." But sleep eluded him, rather he was "continually tossing and turning" at night. He began to get bags under his eyes as he described the "deep darkness on my eyelids." When he did sleep, he was "frightened with dreams" and terrified by visions." His experience was depressing, and possibly traumatic.

His normally rational mind was affected as well. He was a fairly positive person prior to his losses, and initially told his wife that he would not "curse God and die." But the depression robbed even this from him. It began to change the way he thought. Job alluded to potential memory or concentration problems, stating that God had deprived him of "intelligence," which Job clearly had before. You see, Job had much livestock and land. Prior to his calamity, things were going very well for him financially and at least on some level, he must have been able to manage his vast wealth, enlarge his territory, and care for his flocks. But after depression became his companion, he was only able to focus on his deep pain. He moved from complaining to abject bitterness. He stated "I will not restrain my mouth" but will speak in the anguish of my soul. I will complain in the bitterness of myself."

We find that with Job there were periods where he vacillated between hopelessness and hope. Earlier on in his calamity, Job said "though He slay me, I will hope in him" and attempts to encourage himself stating "all the days of my life, I will wait until my change comes." He was the same man who initially knelt to worship God after learning of the death of his children. As time passes, he had periods of doubt where he no longer believed that God would even listen to his voice, and even goes so far as to accuse God of "destroying man's hopes."

Though Job knew that his God had been reliable as a source of hope before, his circumstances seemed to make him question what he thought he knew. He did recover later on reminding himself and his friends that "my redeemer lives" and "even after my skin is destroyed, yet in my flesh I shall see God." Though not an explicit symptom of depression, I have found many patients struggle with similar decision making, vacillating back and forth about how they feel, and what they should do. For many, it takes much effort to make a decision and they would rather others decide on complicated matters and defer decision making. Some question their faith, unsure about the "goodness" of a God who would allow such calamity.

Like Job, many people experience this constellation of symptoms causing some of them to despair life as well. You may have heard the phrase "the patience of Job," but he was human like us, and in his immense struggle, even he experienced suicidal ideation. He described himself as a "bitter soul who longs for death" and asked that God would be willing to "crush" him and cut him off. He wished that there had not been a "day of his birth" and after suffering through his situation, he literally cursed the day he was born. Now, Job did not "read the textbook," so he does not display all of the signs of depression, only most of them. For instance, he does not endorse feelings of guilt or self-blame that can be seen in depression. Rather, he maintains his innocence and vehemently denies any guilt to his friends.

Through Job's story, we get a glimpse of why people who have experienced depression are reluctant to get better for fear of relapse. He actually said, "I rejoice in my sparing pain." Why did he feel this way? In the beginning of his story, Job was told of one calamity, and "before that servant could finish talking, another servant came running to share of another calamity." Have you ever felt like you were just beginning to regain your balance and you get sucker punched with a blow that knocks the wind out of you? Or you were just beginning to see the light at the end of the tunnel and then it got snuffed out. Well, you are not alone. Can you sense it in Job's reactions? Feel his sense of despondency. If you identify with either of the examples I have given thus far, it is likely that you have depression that needs treatment.

What form that treatment takes is up to you to decide. Job went on to have what could loosely be considered "talk therapy," as he was able to verbally process with his friends about his distress. Supportive therapy, Group therapy, and Peer Support have all been utilized to help patients cope with depression. King David used several techniques to get better, including writing and journaling about his experience, using positive affirmations, and forms of exercise. Some of these same techniques may be helpful for you on your journey to health. In the upcoming chapters, we will discuss how to go about seeking treatment, what treatment options are currently available, and how to prevent future recurrences.

CHAPTER 2

Decide If You Want To Get Better Or Not:

Battlefield of the Mind

"Thoughts lead on to purposes; purposes go forth in action; actions form habits; habits decide character; and character fixes our destiny."

- Tyron Edwards

Everyone has their comfortable item of clothing that is threadbare or piece of furniture that is faded and worn. When others look at it, they likely want to cover it, throw it out or burn it. However, to you, it's comfortable and you just cannot see yourself parting with it. We all know what that is like. Depression, oddly enough, is no different. For some, they deal with it for so long, it has become familiar, and even comfortable, to them. If you have been enshrouded with depression, it may have become like a safety blanket. Something that you can turn to again and again. Remember Job's experience. He despaired but also began to find a peculiar mixture of comfort in his depressed state of mind.

Joyce Meyer has written a book about the battle that rages in between your two ears, aptly called "The Battlefield of the Mind." In part, it describes the struggle we each have with thoughts that enter our minds, germinate like seeds, and then direct our feelings and ultimately our actions. Although this is a gross oversimplification of this mental battle, it reminds me of the old Tom and Jerry cartoons I used to watch on Saturday mornings. Tom usually had to decide between doing what he knew was right and what he felt like doing. He knew that what he really felt like doing was not likely to end well for either him or for Jerry. But, he would have a little angel sitting on one of his shoulders and a little devil sitting on the other. Each "thought" tried to affect his feelings and dictate his actions.

For every decision, for every action, we each have to decide what we are going to do with the information that we already have versus the information being presented to us. There are those who have thought they have depression, and are on the fence about talking to someone about it. They fear stigma, or unnecessary loss of time in case there is really not a problem. Do they want to be diagnosed with a mental illness? If so, do they then want the diagnosis? Others with depression may not know that they are being inadequately treated, or undertreated but still war with calling their doctor again to figure out why they are not feeling better. Should they keep taking the medicine the doctor is recommending, or try another method?

Still others have been lifted from the depression with a medicine or therapy for a while. They physically feel like a weight has been lifted off the shoulders. Life seems beautiful again. People seem genuine and caring. They can almost hear an angelic host singing from behind those clouds that actually look like they do have a silver lining. But then the medicine stops working, or they get stuck in therapy, or fired from their job or a host of other life issues. They begin to slip back under that blanket of doom, or worse plummet down into that pit so fast they wonder if that happiness they felt was real or just an illusion. Now, they are torn, between trying to get better and get that life, that hope back again, or giving up altogether.

This is a period that is most concerning to mental health professionals. It is the transition period surrounding either feeling at your worse, or, ironically, beginning to feel better. Much research and lay press attention has been given to the person with depression that has thoughts of self-harm when initially prescribed an antidepressant. The concern is for the one whom medicine and therapy have begun to lift the veil of despondency, who has begun to feel better, and more energetic. It is then that the patient believes that this feeling will not last, and that the hopelessness will return and collide with them like a freight train. The medicine for them, gives them the energy they need to put a plan in place to end their life, but it does not have to be this way. We can begin to do the mental work to defeat depression once and for all.

Regardless of where you fall on your journey, you have to decide if you want to get better. When you feel hopeless, it is difficult to make the decision to leave where you are and go into another unknown. When you see others smiling and living life, you feel that is just unfair. Or worse, as mentioned above, you start feeling better only to return to feeling worse again.

So where do we start? The mind is part of the problem so we will start there. Remember earlier I alluded to the battle going on right now in your mind. We have to train ourselves to evaluate the thoughts that enter and roam freely in our minds. Determine whether it is true or false, positive or negative, encouraging or destructive. Initially, it will be hard work to monitor your thoughts, but it is well worth it. Overtime, it will become like any other routine you have developed.

If you have never dealt with clinical depression, I want you to know there is hope and there is healing. You can be made whole and live your life. If you have been depressed before, you actually have an advantage! Hindsight, like vision, can be 20/20. Having experienced some success before, you know in part, what you need to do to get back to enjoying your life.

From this moment on, choose to intentionally focus on more positive and life giving concepts. No longer let thoughts rent space in your head for free. Choose to assess each thought to determine if it is worthy of living in your head. Ideas and thoughts randomly enter our minds through multiple sources – people, media, and print material, to name a few. Determine if it is positive and useful, or negative and detrimental. If it is positive, do whatever it takes to hold on to it. Write it down. Share it with others. Email it back to yourself. It can positively affect how you live and is a part of the choice to feel better. If it is a negative thought, purpose in your mind how you will discard it. For some, it is as simple as mentally focusing on a different thought. For others, it may mean a systematic process of getting rid of it like you would with any other garbage. This may include writing it down, shredding it, and disposing of it in a trash can.

One of the things I thoroughly enjoy doing with patients is CBT, or Cognitive Behavior Therapy. Introduced by Dr. Aaron Beck in the 1960s, it is a process of reviewing thoughts, feelings, and behavior. I do not know if Dr. Beck knew this or not, but the concept is quite similar to one of King Solomon's wise teachings in his Book of Proverbs. King Solomon came to the conclusion that as a person "thinks in his heart, so is he" in Proverbs 23:7. Think about that for a moment. Thoughts determine the emotions of the "heart", which determine behaviors. So whether you understand this better the way Dr. Beck expressed it or the way King Solomon wrote it, you can use the principle to your advantage.

Sometimes we get too caught up in our feelings, allowing them to rule us rather than the other way around. Feelings can be fickle, and they can be changed. Emotions can be incredibly powerful, but we know that we can affect our feelings by our thoughts. We need to successfully channel our feelings and our emotions. We need to lead them, and not let our feelings or emotions lead us. You can wake up with a thought that you did not get enough rest and feel tired. However, if you have purposefully placed a beautiful motivational picture in your immediate view upon awakening, looking at the picture and reflecting on the positive words can help you choose to change your outlook for the morning.

When I do work in a local jail, one of the things I am incredibly impressed by is how many patients tell me that they are chronically angry. When attempting to process with them, they are often unable to pinpoint a thought related to why they feel angry. They share a situation and immediately jump to the statement "then I got angry." On further questioning, there is often an explanation of the situation or the behaviors, but rarely is there any time given to the preceding thoughts that went through their mind. These are not unintelligent people. However, they have not had practice with identifying the thought that led to the feeling that led to the behavior. They only can tell me their reaction (behavior) in their anger (feeling) that led to a particular behavior.

There are two issues here that I hope you understand. The primary issue in the previous example is skipping past thoughts and moving directly to feelings and behaviors. I find that if we analyze a problem, identify the thoughts that come to mind, and rediscover the underlying feeling, patients can move towards making lasting positive changes in their lives. The other issue seen in the above example is the focusing of so much energy on the emotion of anger that you doom yourself to repeat maladaptive behaviors.

Some of my patients start with an inability to recognize any other emotion but anger. Anger, in all of its forms, is a secondary emotion, but occurs often in many mental illnesses, including depression. We typically call it irritability in depression. It has been taught that other primary emotions, such as hurt, disappointment, and unfairness typically occur first. Hurt can be emotional or physical. Disappointment is usually related to unmet needs and expectations. Unfairness relates to a sense of injustice, or "righteous indignation." Once we identify the reason behind the anger, and identify the primary emotion, it often allows a patient to tap into a wider variety of feelings, and help get to the root of the problem.

Sometimes, in my work with patients I use an emotion wheel or feeling chart, so they can better put into words what's going on in the inside of their mind and their body. There is also a new phrase, "feeling some kind of way" that I did not understand when I first encountered it. This is an allusion to feeling angry, upset, irritated, frustrated, or offended. In essence what it represents is a form of alexithymia. Alexithymia is the inability to put into words what you are feeling. A person struggles to identify or name their feelings. I happen to do a fair amount of trauma work, and from that work, have recognized that when patients experience trauma, they are sometimes unable to access certain feelings or give a name to them. Our brain is so wonderful that it can shield us from very painful emotions.

Many have struggled to remember details of a particularly painful experience and sometimes say they have "blacked out" with no remembrance of their actions. These strong emotions and accompanying memories can prove to be problematic for patients as it can be related to negative and poorly functioning thinking patterns.

Our brains are an incredible network of structures composed of cells that interact with hormones internally and react to the environment around us. In the above example, we discussed how trauma may lead to difficulties accessing emotions buried inside the brain. However, trauma is certainly not the only experience that can affect thoughts and mood. There are several other conditions that not only commonly occur along with depression, but can also cause disordered thinking processes. We will shortly discuss them, but I mention them here because they can seemingly make the process of monitoring your thoughts more difficult. But if you educate yourself about them, it will not be as difficult as you think. For each of these disorders, I will explain how they can affect your thinking, and how you can guard your thoughts against them.

Many of my patients struggle with both depression and anxiety. I have often seen that where depression is driving, anxiety is often a passenger. However, anxiety disorders are even more insidious and many people adapt to them to the point that they often do not recognize their thoughts as being anxious or their bodily reactions as being related to the anxiety. For example, many patients with Generalized Anxiety Disorder worry about a variety of things and have difficulties controlling their worry. Many have anxious thoughts all throughout the day and misinterpret bodily reactions. When doing relaxation activities with them, they struggle to relax. They may think this is "normal" for them, and sometimes that they are diagnosed with another illness. Unfortunately, anxiety disorders can also occur with or worsen other medical illnesses, such as high blood pressure, reflux disease, and certain types of headaches. Patients can be taught to recognize anxious thoughts and their associated physical symptoms so that they can retrain the brain.

Chronic pain is another co-occurring disorder. Many patients deal with acute pain following an injury or procedure, such as surgery. Unfortunately, a patient's pain can transition from acute pain, typically occurring within days to weeks, to chronic pain, which occurs from months to years. Chronic pain is a complex condition, sometimes beginning with an acute process, but other times, it develops so silently there is no easy disease process to identify initially. I have had many patients who have been given opiate medicines by a physician for acute pain, but then continue these medicines for chronic pain. Scientifically, we know this does not work long term.

There is a vicious cycle that begins. When you are in pain, you typically feel worse in terms of your mood. When your mood is low, you want to do less, both physically and mentally. You do less, which deconditions your body, leading to less energy and typically less motivation. Physically as you are no longer able to do many of the things to which you were accustomed, so your mood becomes even lower. Before long, you become discouraged in addition to being deconditioned. You are now less able to do as much physically or mentally and the cycle continues. This pattern creates a connection in the brain between your physical pain and emotional pain. This is why opiate medicines designed to address acute physical pain do little for long term chronic pain. Of note, chronic pain is a combination of both physical and emotional pain types. If we intervene and focus our mental energy on breaking all aspects of the pain cycle, we can overcome it.

Our discussion on depression and chronic pain leads us to another common co-occurring disorder - Addiction. Patients, who start out in treatment with providers, can begin using legally obtained opiate medication inappropriately and then transition to use of illegal substances. The majority of heroin users began using legally prescribed prescription opiate medication. Whether it started as treatment for physical pain or emotional pain, many of my patients turned to non-prescription substances to "self-medicate" or "numb the pain." Some use alcohol or drugs, while others use gambling or sex. In 2016, Surgeon General Murthy released the report "Facing Addiction in America," outlining this process and making a call for change in the way this mental illness is viewed.

I have some patients tell me they would rather "self-medicate" with "legal" substances, but what they are often missing is the need to get to the root of the problem and not only treat symptoms. Addictions, like the other conditions we discussed, change the way your brain functions. Substances "hijack" the brain, becoming more valuable than things we need to survive long term, like food and sex (e.g. relationships). Conquering addiction begins with having your mind firmly fixed on getting free from it.

I have introduced the need to begin monitoring your thoughts and see the connection to your feelings, or mood, and your current behaviors. In the next chapter, we will discuss several treatment options. It is my hope that you have now made the choice to move forward in finding options that will work for you.

CHAPTER 3

How to Get Better Faster:

Developing Your System

"Sound advice is a beacon, good teaching is a light, discipline is a life path"

- King Solomon

In Chapter 2, we discussed how important it was to make a conscious decision that you wanted to get better. Congratulations on your decision to move forward. Now, let's get to work. When I was in medical school, I remember feeling overwhelmed by the volume of information that I was expected to understand and retain. In order to succeed, I learned two things fairly quickly. I had to develop an efficient system for learning and if there were things I did not know, I had to know how to access the correct information with as little effort as possible so that I could expend my energy on the most important things – passing my exams and taking care of patients.

My system started with a grasp of the major organizational structure of how the human body worked. I built a scaffold, or skeleton, in my mind, and started hanging more and more ideas on this scaffold, similar to the way muscles and skin are layered on the human body. Though details are always intriguing, I had to force myself to learn the basic information first, so that I had a good understanding of what was going on as learning adds on over time. Once I had the basic fundamentals down pat, there were still gaps in knowledge as there is simply too much new information made available every day for one person to grasp it all. I typically worked with small groups to collectively share information. We were accountable to each other, and as one learned, we all learned and ultimately succeeded in reaching our goal of completing medical school.

For you to get the best results in terms of overcoming depression, defining your goal and creating a system to get there will be necessary. My goal for you is not just symptom reduction, but complete eradication of the illness of depression. Together, you and I will discuss the system that you will use to find success, but we will start with the bare bones of treatment options. Then we will add details in later chapters. Furthermore, if there are remaining knowledge gaps, I will share resources that you can turn to where others, who are on the journey with you, can share their collective wisdom. Our scaffold begins with your belief system, and since this is like the skeleton of the body, it is the weightiest portion to read and gain understanding. We will then move on to writing down your goals and monitoring your moods. A list of non-medicine options to include in your arsenal against depression will be provided. In the next chapter, we will discuss medical options, including medicines and other treatments.

Your Scaffold: Your Faith Belief System

"Just because we happen not to have actually seen something with our own two little winkies, we think it is not existing."

-The BFG, Roald Dahl

I am a movie and music person, so you will see allusions to both in this chapter. In the movie Akeelah and the Bee, Akeelah is a gifted speller who is mentored by a tough, but caring coach for the National Scripp's Spelling Bee. Her goal is winning the competition, but the odds are stacked against her. When she first meets her coach, it takes him a while to help her believe that winning the championship is an option for her. Despite this, she begins to do well, but struggles when her coach is unable to help her prepare further because of his own limitations. However, he does not leave her helpless. He teaches her that others in her life can support her in meeting her goal. Before his initial departure, her coach was reading, quizzing, and testing her on cards for spelling and origin of words. After his teaching, Akeelah learns that others can quiz and encourage her to reach her goal. She gets help from her mother, brother, peers, and neighbors. She found her tribe of helpers, her support system. However, as mentioned earlier, her support system was not the first part of her system that needed to be developed. Her success story starts with what she believed she was able to do.

Let's begin with a discussion of your belief system and how it is affecting depression. As a Christian, I have a Christian world view and, thus, my faith belief system comes from the Bible. Even if you are an atheist and you believe that there is no God, or agnostic and you are not quite sure if there is a God, this section still applies to you. Regardless of what you choose to believe, you have some belief system. What you believe will in part dictate your success.

I remember reading the story of the *Little Engine That Could*, when I was a child. The Little Engine was smaller than the rest of the train that he had to pull up a steep hill, but because he believed he could pull it, he did. He reminded himself as he was chugging up the hill, "I think I can, I think I can." His thoughts and his beliefs, both later translated into words, were remarkably powerful in helping him achieve his reality. Thinking positive thoughts and speaking positive words are both very powerful principles. I would consider both universal principles, or laws, that transcend religion and culture. Whether we believe in them or not, certain universal laws apply to each of us. For instance, there is the Law of Gravity. Before we knew anything about the Law of Gravity, we were still subject to it. If I threw an apple into the air, and stood under it, even if I did not believe in the law, I would still get hit in the head with the apple.

Warren Buffett, Oprah Winfrey, and Bill Gates are some of the wealthiest people in the world. Believe it or not, they practice biblical principles every day and may not even know it. There is a biblical law that if a person "gives abundantly, they will receive abundantly," according to 2 Corinthians 9:6. These three people are very abundant givers, and cannot seem to give their money away faster than what it returns to them. They may or may not believe in the Bible, but they benefit from this biblical law. As author Andy Stanley has said, "You do not have to believe the Bible to read it." Likewise, you do not have to believe in the Bible to benefit from the universal principles it contains.

I firmly believe that anyone that wants to be better can get better. They just need the right resources. The main resource is hope. Even if I believe you can get better, you have to believe you can get better. You have to have something to hope for, something to push you forward towards your goal. What do you hope for? Do you have hope that you can get better? For your children? Your family? Your memories of what it used to be like when you were happier, healthier? Whatever it is, write it down. For the Christian, remember that Christ is hope. But Christians are not inhuman. They suffer loss and hardship like everybody else. Regardless of your faith, you sometimes need a professional to help get you to the place where you can believe you can feel better again. Mental health professionals can serve as a bridge to help you access hope until you can find the path for yourself. So, whether your hope comes directly through your faith, or through another means, recognize your motivation for tackling the problem. Please write it down and place it in a prominent place that you will see at least once a day. In the upcoming sections, there will be many opportunities for you to make more decisions, including what you will choose to believe for your health. For now, you can borrow from my belief that you can be in good health and free from depression.

Thinking in Terms of Systems

In the movie analogy given above, Akeelah had a system. For her to learn and retain the information she needed for the National Scripps Spelling Bee, she utilized a way of keeping letters in her head and had an innate sense of rhythm. As her coach explained, many other students had some type of system for keeping track of the letters they needed to spell words. To keep her rhythm and her momentum while spelling words, Akeelah used everything from tapping the side of her leg to jumping rope as a part of her system. As mentioned before, you need a system in place so that you can achieve your goal. You and your mental health professionals are a team that can come up with a treatment plan *and* a system for following that plan that works uniquely for you.

First, let's build your team. Let's go back to the cancer example from Chapter 1. If you were diagnosed with breast cancer, you will likely have several providers on your team, each doing different jobs. The Primary Care Provider (PCP) helps with initial diagnosis of the cancer and referral to specialists. A Surgeon may remove diseased breast tissue containing cancer through surgery. A Pathologist, or doctor that studies tissues and cells of the body, will look intently at the breast and surrounding tissue under a microscope to make sure the Surgeon got all of the visible cancer cells out. One type of cancer doctor, a Medical Oncologist may recommend chemotherapy, or a medicine in a pill to get rid of any cells that are too small to be seen. You may also have a different type of cancer doctor, a Radiation Oncologist, use a special machine to target the cancer cells and destroy them with radiation. In addition to the doctors, other professionals are also necessary, including but not limited to Nutritional support and Case management. Often, Complementary and Alternative Medicines, or CAM, is utilized. A CAM provider may recommend herbal remedies or use of essential oils. The patient with cancer has developed a team that helps care for them.

You will also need to develop your professional mental health team, if you have not already done so. As in the cancer example, this typically starts with your Primary Care Provider who can help with diagnosis of depression. At this point, some Christians are particularly reluctant to seek mental health care. Unfortunately, due to the particular stigma related to mental illness in the church, many feel uncomfortable seeking help from their Pastor or local congregation. I have seen much written about how all depression is demonic, and I disagree with this. This makes it difficult for many patients to get the help they need. If this is something you have encountered, this book can help you find a safe place to help you meet your needs. Seeking treatment from a licensed Christian counselor may be a good place to start. After entering treatment, you may be referred to a therapist, a Psychiatrist, or another specialist depending on associated symptoms you have. Case management, Nutrition support, and an Herbal medicine specialist may be helpful as well.

Once you start building your team, share openly what you are dealing with so that they can help you decide on what the best treatment is for you. Your team will share additional ideas about what system based approaches may help in your unique situation. In thinking about Akeelah, the system that she used helped her achieve her goal of winning a National spelling bee. Now, your system is going to help you achieve your goal of overcoming depression.

Make Self-care A Priority

If you have ridden in a plane, you would have heard the steward or stewardess give the caution that if there is a loss of cabin pressure, an oxygen mask will come down from the ceiling. They then give an instruction that is counterintuitive to every parent or caregiver on the plane. They tell you to first put the oxygen mask on yourself, then put it on the person needing assistance. Why? With the loss of oxygen, if you struggle to put it on your loved one first, you may pass out before you are able to complete the task leaving your children, aging parent, or disabled neighbor with no source of help.

Determine now, before distraction sets in, that you will make your mental health a priority. Before your family, your livelihood, or any other responsibility that you have, self-care needs to be an important priority. You cannot give to others what you do not have. Many have used the analogy of a full bucket that can then be used to pour into others. Self-care is doing what you need to keep your bucket relatively full. If you are unhealthy, that will spill over to all of these other areas. Focus on being healthy. Self-care is not selfish. It is likely the most unselfish thing that you could do to make sure you are functioning to the best of your capacity. You may need help with carving out time for self-care. There are many resources available to help with self-care. Several are listed at the end of book in the Resources section, but to get you started let's make a matrix to help you work through now what needs to be a priority and what does not.

Former U.S. President Dwight D. Eisenhower's Decision Matrix was said to have helped him in his successful career. The one you will make will be similar to the matrix table labeled below with

IMPORTANT at the top and URGENT on the left hand side. Start filling in the box as outlined below, listing things that are both URGENT and IMPORTANT, IMPORTANT but NOT URGENT, URGENT but NOT IMPORTANT, and NOT IMPORTANT and NOT URGENT. Once you have completed this, immediately purpose to get rid of, or at the least put out of your mind, things that are NOT IMPORTANT and NOT URGENT. These are usually distractions. Now, move on to the things that are IMPORTANT and URGENT. Here is where your priority is and why self-care is vital. You need the bulk of your energy and to be your best self for these things. Things that are URGENT, but NOT IMPORTANT are things that you will need to delegate to others if you can. This is where your Support Team, discussed below, will begin to help. That is perfectly fine since it is okay to ask for help. When addressing the IMPORTANT but NOT URGENT box, it is helpful to set up reminders so that these things are not forgotten, but taken care of as time and energy permit.

	Important	Not Important
Urgent	Important and Urgent	Urgent but Not Important
Not Urgent	Important but Not Urgent	Not Important and Not Urgent

Write Your Health Vision

Akeelah's goal was winning the championship. Your goal is no less glorious. It is victory over depression and your treatment plan solidifies your goal. Saying that you will no longer be depressed is helpful, but it can be even more specific. Think of it like you are trying to decide how you want to run and finish a race. Which race are you running? A 100 meter dash? A 5 kilometer? A marathon? Determining what race you will run will dictate how you will need to train to finish your race. What is your goal for finishing? It takes one mindset to simply cross the finish line injury free and an entirely different mindset to finish with a bronze, silver, or gold medal. Like any goal, your depression treatment goal should be specific and measurable. For example, reducing your symptoms of depression by half over a two month period as measured by a Depression screen is a specific and measurable goal that can be discussed with your provider. For now, start with writing down what your goal is as well as the symptoms that you wish to target initially. Take this with you when you visit your provider so that, together, you can create your health vision.

Creating Your Support System

When I counsel clients, I often have them complete a Safety Treatment Plan, not necessarily because they are suicidal. Rather it is for them to see on paper, in black and white what their resources are and who is a part of their support system. Included is always their professional mental health team, serving in the same capacity as the coach for Akeelah. But like the coach, these folks are not always fully available 24 hours a day, 7 days a week. Like Akeelah, your support team will also include other people in your life that care about your goal. Sometimes your friend is a great shoulder to cry on and can be listed as a support. Other times, you may choose a different friend with whom you would not necessarily share certain details of your life, but is a great resource for getting you out of the house and distracting you from your problems. That is why people that you can talk to as well as those who can provide distraction are listed in many treatment plans.

Some patients are reluctant to complete a plan outlining their support system, as they feel alone with the exception of professionals. That may be true right now, but it certainly does not have to stay that way. Social media has drastically changed how the world connects to each other. I recommend in the Resources section organizational sites that contain positive and inspiring content. Some provide access to an online supportive environment while others can help you connect with people who have similar experiences. Podcasts can be helpful to listen to stories of how others have overcome depression as well as other educational content. Look for articles and posts that are inspirational and uplifting.

Monitoring Moods

In Chapter 2, I introduced the concept of monitoring your thoughts, feelings, and behavior. Dr. Beck created the tracking system that most people use with Cognitive Behavior Therapy. Other therapies certainly exist and are helpful, but most are based in some ways, on the principles Dr. Beck outlined in his book. When working with a patient, I explain the relationship between the three components in the following way. I want to take you to lunch, but we are meeting someone there and that person is 15 minutes late. That is the situation we are dealing with and this does not change. However, what you know about the person we are meeting does change.

In our first example, the person is someone you know and they are known to be chronically late. What thoughts go through your mind? How do you feel? What do you do? Well, your thoughts are your cognition, your feeling is your mood, and what you do is your behavior. In our second example, the person we are meeting is also someone you know, but they are normally quite punctual. Now, what thoughts go through your mind? What are your feelings about this person's late arrival? What do you do? One more example. Let's say we are meeting someone we do not know. They are a friend of a friend, and we have no prior experience with them in terms of their reliability. What do you think if this person arrives late? How is your mood? What do you do this time?

There are several points for this illustration. The situation did not change in the above example. It was a neutral and common occurrence to which many can relate. I want you to notice that your thoughts, feelings, and behavior are likely different based on your experience with the person. Our experience drives much of how you perceive the world around you and how you then react to it. As we discussed previously, the brain sets up systems automatically to guard us from emotional pain. If based on your past experience, you have learned people are hurtful and untrustworthy, even when presented with a seemingly "neutral" situation, you may think and react differently from someone else without your baseline of experiences.

We are creatures of habit, and we will tend to slip into the same thinking patterns again and again. Going through this process of monitoring thoughts, feelings, and behavior will first help you see how you currently think. Then, you can go through the process of checking your thoughts for truth, challenging thinking that is untrue, and finally addressing possible alternate behaviors. Over time, this process causes changes in your brain that are similar to what is achieved with medicines, and more importantly, may be more permanent. Think about that. A permanent change for the better. Isn't that worth making the effort?

Playing Mind Games: Mindfulness and Meditation

We have family game nights in our home, and even though there is stiff competition, it's an enjoyable experience all done in love. There are not a lot of rules, but one that is strictly enforced is no electronics at the table. Electronics become a distraction that pulls the members of the family away from our primary objective, which is enjoying our time together. We try to be mindful and focus on each other, rather than our cell phone, the television, or the computer.

Mindfulness is not a new concept, and in this section, I am simply talking about being focused on the moment. We are such a busy, modern society. We often rush from one event to the next, barely taking time to enjoy anything. It leads to discontentment and a lack of gratitude for the good things we already have. Taking the time to reflect on the positive things in your life can be helpful. Developing an "attitude of gratitude" is both wholesome in life and abundantly necessary in conquering depression. As I mentioned earlier, King David seemed to have a tried and true method for dealing with his depressed mood. In Psalm after Psalm, he displays a similar pattern. He admits to his feelings of despondency, sometimes lamenting the circumstances that brought him to his current state. But, the reader quickly sees him shift his focus from his current state to an attribute of God, such as faithfulness or strength. By the end of the Psalm, King David is now expressing gratitude, and, at least for the moment, the depression is forgotten.

Meditation is a popular method for improved mental clarity and health. Again, in this section I am using a very simple definition. To meditate means to ponder, to give sustained attention to something. If you are in school studying for an exam, if you do not meditate on the material for an extended period of time to understand it, it is likely that your test grade will reflect that you do not know the material well. When overcoming depression, you need to meditate on positive and encouraging material. In Chapter 6, quotes and scriptures are provided to help with positive things on which you can focus. Christians are actually encouraged to meditate on the scriptures many times in the Bible. Focusing on nature can also be a helpful guide for positivity (see below). I do not recommend clearing the mind of all thoughts because this leaves too much room to slip back into the habit of focusing again on the problem of depression.

When I have a patient who is interested in it, I provide them with a Prescription based on the author Paul's book to the Philippians in Chapter 4. In verse 8, he tells you what to focus on in meditation. He tells us to focus only on things that are true, honest, just, pure, lovely, good, virtuous, and things that people would praise. This is a great way to shift your focus from your problem to contentment and help you get towards gratitude. Before moving on to the next section, make a list of each one thing from the above eight focus points. To help you there is a chart below with examples from nature.

Examples of Things to Focus On	
True	Mockingbirds
Honest	Water
Just	The Ocean
Pure	Gold, Snow in the Alaskan Wilderness
Lovely	Botanical Gardens
Good	Sunrise and Sunset
Virtuous	Doves
Praise worthy	Redwoods of California

Visualization and Film

"Movies touch our hearts and awaken our vision, and change the way we see things. They take us out to other places, they open doors and minds." - Martin Scorsese

Imagery is powerful and can be used to improve your mood instantly. Think how you can be affected by a photo sent to you by a friend that instantly lifts your spirits. Many pictures paired with inspirational words grace both businesses and homes. Books and poetry invoke imagery and take us to places both distant and near. Think of Robert Frost's classic, "The Road Not Taken." We can see the fork in the road in our minds as he describes, and translate it to the crossroads in our lives when it comes to the major decisions we have to make. Film is a very powerful form of imagery with its combination of pictures, words, and music. Who has not been moved by the combination of a beautiful musical score coupled with brilliant acting?

For a moment, we can do a bit of guided imagery, similar to what I would do in my office with patients. In office, I will pull up on the computer a picture of something that they find peaceful. I have them close their eyes, if they feel comfortable with this, and begin with three deep breaths. Most of us do not breathe as deeply throughout the day as we should. Again, our fast pace is reflected even here, as we move, and breathe, shallowly throughout life. So, practicing the deep breathing helps increase oxygen to the brain and slowly begins the process of relaxing other portions of the body. If they wish, we then add a bit of Progressive Muscle Relaxation and have them slowly tense various muscle groups as they breathe in and relax their muscles as they exhale out.

Finally, when they are more relaxed, I have them recall the image they see on the screen and imagine themselves in that special, peaceful place. I have the patient explain to me how they are experiencing their five senses, both in their imagination and physically in the room. This helps them to stay both engaged in the experience and be "grounded" in the room with me. What I mean by that is patients with trauma may have a tendency to dissociate and wander mentally. I "keep them in the room" by using taste, touch, sight, hearing, and smell so that they enjoy the relaxing experience without drifting mentally into a potentially trauma induced state. For example, if we are on the beach, they share with me the seagulls they see, the sound of the ocean they hear, the salt water they can taste and smell, and the wind that breezes past them.

Hormonal

While we will talk about medicines in the next part of this chapter, there are many activities that you can do to help increase some of the same hormones that medicines will increase. The next two subsections discuss quick things you can do to help alter your mood and begin to change your brain.

Music and laughter are discussed first, followed by exercise. Nutrition is discussed in Chapter 4.

Music

"My heart, which is so full to overflowing, has often been solaced and refreshed by music when sick and weary."

- Martin Luther

We are so impacted by the spoken word, particularly when put to music. Music does not have to be accompanied by words to move us. Just listen to Itzhak Perlman play Vivaldi's *Four Seasons Spring* or Dizzy Gillespie's *Bebop*. How can music like this be used to our advantage? Listening to positive, upbeat music instantly lifts the spirits. There is a local radio station that brands itself as being "positive and encouraging." Be purposeful in choosing the music that you surround yourself. Let it be positive and encouraging, particularly if you know that you have struggled with depression in the past. It does not matter the genre. Classical, Country, Jazz, Gospel, Opera, Celtic, Hip Hop, Rock and Roll or Rhythm and Blues. Yes, even the Blues can be uplifting, in both the rhythm as well as the lyrics. Die hard Blues fans can find solace in B. B. King's *Feel like a million* and Eric Clapton's *Change the World*, both of which have positive themes.

You do have to be careful about the lyrics to which you listen. I have seen patient's present in clinic in distress and we were able, in part, to trace it back to certain types of music to which they listened. Did music alone begin a spiral towards depression? No, but it was a key factor in shifting their mood and in clinic we had an intelligent discussion about the powerful connection of music to trigger an emotionally charged memory. Begin now taking stock of the music you listen to and how the music makes you feel. Then challenge yourself to still listen to the same genre, but focus on songs that have more positive lyrics. Record the effect on your mood. It will be interesting to see if there is a difference.

Making Merry

"From there to here, from here to there, funny things are everywhere."

One fish, Two fish, Red fish, Blue fish by Dr. Seuss

Laughter is good medicine for the soul and much has been written about its positive effect on mood. Watching old cartoons, television shows, and standup comedians is one way to tickle your funny bone. Reading comic strips are another great tool to lift your mood almost immediately. Jeff Larson has a wonderful comic strip called *The Back Pew*. It's very funny, uplifting, and encouraging. YouTube and GodTube can both be good resources for the funny and the inspiring. Almost anything that will put a smile on your face can have immediate and long lasting benefits. Sit and think of a funny conversation you have had with a friend or a funny comic that you heard. Even years later, the memory can still bring a smile. Chapter 7 goes more into the science behind this.

Education

Depression and Diabetes have much in common. Besides both starting with the letter D, they both cause significant morbidity and mortality. They can cause complications to your health if not treated appropriately, but the two medical conditions have recognized treatment algorithms that do work. They can both be completely treated using a team approach. Interestingly, both of them have significant stigma attached to them. Many people believe all people who have diabetes are obese. They also can occur together as many people with depression also have an underlying medical issue.

Unlike depression, we have made more progress with diabetes in terms of stigma, treatments, and Diabetes Education. Diabetes Educators are trained to help patients with diabetes understand their illness and make changes so that they can reach their goal of managing and potentially eliminating the diagnosis. It is not often recommended that patients with depression see a Depression Educator, like we would with diabetes.

When a pill is prescribed for treatment of depression, providers and patients consider the medicine's ability to work, be tolerated, and risk of side effects and potential interactions. Well, if psycho-education about depression were a pill, I can tell you that risks of common side effects like nausea, diarrhea, constipation, headache, dizziness, weight gain, and rash are non-existent. It is efficacious and tolerable. There are no known risks, but interactions, I am happy to say, are bountiful. When education is combined with action, there is no end to the number of benefits that can occur. Education can come from many reliable sources and I would encourage you to take advantage of those from reputable mental health organizations, therapists, and, in many cases, trained peer counselors. While there is a larger list in the Resources Section, the National Alliance on Mental Illness (NAMI) and Mental Health America (MHA) are both credible places to start or narrow your search to meet your unique needs. As noted in a previous section, NAMI also offers opportunity to connect with peer counselors that provide credibility as they are on the journey along with, and often a bit ahead of you.

Exercise

According to the Physical Activity Guidelines for Americans, it is recommended that adults receive "at least 150 minutes of moderate intensity" or 75 minutes of "vigorous intensity aerobic activity" a week. This translates into 22 minutes a day for six days a week or 25 minutes a day for seven days a week for moderate exercises. Do you have 20 minutes out of your 1,440 minutes a day that you plan to do some type of physical activity? You can do any type of exercise that you enjoy. While it is recommended that muscle and bone strengthening occur at least three days a week, the other four are free for you to do whatever you like. For my elderly or chronic pain patients, I recommend starting out very slowly, typically with chair aerobics or walking. There are many of both types of exercise examples on the internet.

Even with intense pain issues, you can do something to begin reconditioning your body. Physical therapy can be good places to start if you are deconditioned. If you have a gym membership, group exercise fosters accountability among others who frequent the group. If you do not have a membership, YouTube is full of videos of group exercise classes. I often recommend Zumba because it's similar to dancing, which many people enjoy. Online classes and social media support groups are also becoming more popular and available.

Start with something you enjoy and that will work for your schedule. If my patient is a busy corporate executive who works from 6:00 a.m. until 3 p.m., and generally goes home to spend time with his wife and children, he may be quite reluctant to go to the gym to exercise. I will likely recommend a type of medicine to start helping with depression if his depression is moderate to severe. We would discuss a system for taking medicines at a time of day that he will remember and not have unwanted side effects. Then, the recommendation for him is to exercise with his family with activities that encourage bonding, like walking, biking, or motion-based video gaming. Movement video games such as the Sports editions of the *Wii* and *Kinect* systems as well as dancing games such as *Just Dance* and *Dance Dance Revolution* can be attractive to all age groups, from toddlers to teens and beyond.

Thus far, we have covered several things that can have an immediate impact on your mood and your health. While there are many options in addition to the above for beginning your journey towards improved mental health, start with one or two of these today, then modify as needed. In the next chapter, we will talk about both conventional and non-conventional medicine options for the treatment of depression.

CHAPTER 4

Medicines and Treatments

"Come on in the room. Jesus is my doctor. He writes down all of my 'scriptions, and He gives me all of my medicines in the room"

– Old Negro Spiritual

As mentioned previously, depression can be a time limited illness that does not recur for many people. A medicine may not be necessary for relief of the illness, although medicine typically lessens both the severity and length of most illnesses, depression included. As addressed in Chapter 3, many patients find symptom relief with non-medical options, such as with music and laughter. I do not pretend to know for which patients only the "tincture of time" is needed just as I do not inherently know for whom multiple medicine trials with more extensive treatment will be required. I only know that the process of coming alongside a patient in their suffering and helping to provide relief from their misery is a part of the art of medicine.

In this section we will discuss treatments in both traditional, or Allopathic medicine, as well as natural medicine, sometimes referred to as holistic medicine. For the sake of this section, nutrition, herbal remedies, and essential oils are included as many things that are either ingested internally or applied externally for the purpose of promoting health and wellness and can cause harmful effects if used inappropriately. As such, they should be a part of the conversation you have with you healthcare provider.

I have been asked by fellow Christians about the preference for prayer alone versus taking a medicine along with prayer. Interestingly, this question is asked of many illnesses, not just depression. While I will specifically address depression as it is the subject we are discussing, some of this information can apply to other illness and diseases as well. Unfortunately, there is a teaching in some religions that mental illness is a weakness and that people of faith who became depressed lack moral strength or faith in God to heal. I would be remiss as both a psychiatrist and a Christian if I said this attitude is acceptable. Most assuredly, it is not acceptable.

Many patients, Christians included, can become ill with a variety of ailments and may need proper medical treatment. It would be uncommon to tell a person with a severely infected tooth not to allow the dentist to treat it, or to tell a person with breast cancer not to consider surgery. Yet, I commonly hear people profess fear of seeking help, particularly when they believe their faith will be questioned by others. While I have seen miraculous things, I also believe that a creative God has given "witty inventions and ideas" to doctors for the purpose of healing. Did you know that the modern day symbol of medicine, the Caduceus, is based on a Biblical story of healing in the book of Exodus?

Why do I as a Christian and a Psychiatrist recommend medicines? Jesus, the Great Physician, used a medicine to heal people. In the book of John Chapter 9, the story is told of a blind man who desired to be healed. Jesus knelt down, spat on the ground, and made a compound of the saliva and dirt. He then placed it on the man's eyes and the man was healed from his blindness. Jesus was very powerful; he could just speak to the wind and the waves and they did exactly as He asked. He spoke to or simply touched many and healed them. He did not need to use anything other than Himself. But, in this story of the blind man, He chose to use something external to Himself. He is called the Balm in Gilead. What is a balm? My elders used to call it a salve, or an ointment, or even liniment. It was a medicine used in ancient times to promote healing, particularly in wound care. What is a medicine? It's a mixture or compound that we either take internally or externally. I do not deny the benefit of the power of medicine, natural or synthetic. In the example above, Jesus himself used both prayer and medicine to get the result of healing.

Currently, there is no medicine that exists today that is completely without side effects or potential interactions with other medicines. Even an over-the-counter aspirin can create problems if taken inappropriately or with other medicines that add to its effects. I tell patients that when they are taking a medicine that has to go in the mouth and come out the bottom, it can cause problems all along the way. The body is looking at the medicine as a foreign substance and has to decide what to do with it. When the medicine hits the stomach, you may experience nausea, and as it passes along the gut, diarrhea or constipation, depending on how your body reacts to the new substance. Once it is in the bloodstream, the medicine has to be broken down and finally cross into the brain. You may experience nausea again because there is a nausea center in the brain. Like any medicine that has an effect on the brain, you may experience dizziness, lightheadedness, or headaches when the medicine is initially started. These general side effects tend to last several days, and then resolve with continued medicine use. This is true of pharmaceutical grade medicines as well as herbals, vitamins, and supplements

Allopathic Medicine

There is evidence to support use of psychotherapy as opposed to medications for some forms of depression. The brain changes that occur with psychotherapy are similar to medicine in mild to moderate depression. Adequate therapy does involve a time investment, and depending on the therapist, homework assignments as well. However, the internal side effects that can be experienced with a medication do not occur with psychotherapy. However, psychotherapy is not without some risk. Patients, particularly those with significant trauma history, can experience temporary worsening of some symptoms as information is process in therapy. Some patients are wary of engaging in therapy due to a previous negative experience or perceived time limitations. Just as each person is unique, so are therapists. You are encouraged to select a therapist with care, and if you are not comfortable, let that therapist know and then find a different therapist.

Some patients desire to begin use of a medicine in addition to or instead of therapy. There are several classes of antidepressants and your health care provider can help guide you through the selection process. The initial antidepressants that were made in pill format were the Tricyclic antidepressants (TCAs), and contrary to popular belief, these are very effective medications. However, they did have some concerning side effects and are not used quite as widely as when they first came on the market in the 1950s. They tend to cause sedation and weight gain; patients with heart and liver problems need to use them with caution.

The most popular antidepressants today are the SSRIs, or Selective Serotonin Reuptake inhibitors. The first of these was Prozac, or Fluoxetine, which was created in 1987. That was followed by others you see in the table below. SSRIs tend to cause less side effects compared to TCAs, and are often considered first line treatment for many mood disorders, including depression. These medications can be very helpful for depression, and in some cases, anxiety disorders. However, they all tend to have different indications, or illnesses for which the FDA, or Food and Drug Administration, approves them. For example, Fluvoxamine (Luvox) is FDA approved for treatment of Major Depressive

Disorder and Obsessive Compulsive Disorder, which is an anxiety disorder.

Other antidepressant medications include the SNRIs, or Selective Norepinephrine Reuptake Inhibitors and NDRIs, Norepinephrine Dopamine Reuptake Inhibitors. The SNRIs have been known to help with pain and mood. Duloxetine (Cymbalta) is FDA approved for treatment of Chronic Pain Disorders. Bupropion is a NDRI that can help with sexual side effects sometimes caused by other antidepressants, and may help with concentration. It has also been used to reduce cravings for substances, such as tobacco. The Atypical antidepressants can be used for a variety of symptoms that can occur in depression. For example, Trazodone is often used for insomnia. Monoamine Oxidase Inhibitors, or MAOIs, such as Phenelzine, are typically used less commonly due to need for very strict diet related to interactions with certain foods as well as other medicines. Please see the tables below for more examples of antidepressants.

Serotonin Selective Reuptake Inhibitor
Citalopram (Celexa)
Escitalopram (Lexapro)
Fluoxetine (Prozac)
Fluvoxamine (Luvox)
Paroxetine (Paxil)
Sertraline (Zoloft)

Serotonin Norepinephrine Reuptake Inhibitor
Desvenlafaxine (Pristiq, Khedezla)
Duloxetine (Cymbalta)
Levomilnacipran (Fetzima)
Venlafaxine (Effexor)

Tricyclic Antidepressants
Amitriptyline (Elavil)
Desipramine (Norpramin)
Doxepin (Sinequan)
Imipramine (Tofranil)
Nortriptyline (Pamelor)
Protriptyline (Vivactil)
Trimipramine (Surmontil)

Monoamine Oxidase Inhibitors
Isocarboxazid (Marplan)
Phenelzine (Nardil)
Selegiline (Emsam)
Tranylcypromine (Parnate)

Norepinephrine and Dopamine Reuptake Inhibitor
Bupropion (Wellbutrin, Aplenzin)

Atypical Antidepressants
Mirtazapine (Remeron)
Trazodone (Oleptro)
Vilazodone (Viibryd)
Vortioxetine (Brintellix)

When selecting a medicine, patients should have a conversation about the benefits, risks, and interactions of medicines. Some patients are nervous about starting a medicine, but it is uncommon for most patients to experience side effects outside of those discussed earlier in the chapter. Patients are often more fearful of the prospect of side effects they have read or heard about in the package insert. Let me offer a few recommendations. Prior to leaving your provider's office, openly discuss any concerns you may have. When picking up medicine at the pharmacy or formulary, speak to the pharmacist about information from the insert that is of particular concern. If you still have questions, share this with the provider who gave you the prescription or formulary. Consider taking the medicine for at least three days if you do experience mild side effects as these are likely to stop after a few days.

There are a few serious concerns that are worth mentioning in this section about antidepressants. Recently some patients have expressed concern about an antidepressant Black Box Warning. This is when the FDA labels a medicine for particular caution. All antidepressants have this warning due to concern for increased suicidal ideation and behaviors, particularly among adolescents. Please note that in the analysis of multiple studies done thus far, there have been reports of a small risk of increased thoughts of suicide within the initial period of use of the medicine. The reason for this is unknown, but as mentioned in Chapter 1, changes in mood, including mood and energy improvement can place some patients at risk for self-harm. Because of these concerns, there should be a conversation between you and your doctor about how medicine could affect you. Most patients do not experience thoughts of self-harm, but knowing what the FDA label means can reduce fear of the medicine.

Serotonin Syndrome is another serious medical condition that some patients or family members raise concerns about. This can occur when there is too much of the Serotonin hormone in your system. When I describe this to patients, I explain to them that they may experience sudden flu-like symptoms. You may feel hot and achy with a fever, as well as headache, confusion and restlessness. However, this typically occurs within hours of taking medicines that increase Serotonin. Serotonin level can also be affected by other medicines besides antidepressants. Discontinuation Syndrome can occur with certain medicines that are not weaned slowly enough. Symptoms are not limited only to antidepressants; this can occur with many different types of medicines that are stopped too quickly causing your brain and body to protest in various ways, depending on the medicine.

Once you have begun taking a medicine, it may work quite well for you. However, one medicine alone may not be effective. Another antidepressant, particularly one from another class, may be added. If this is not effective, a different type of medicine may be used to augment, or add to, the antidepressant. As there is a known connection between abnormal thyroid function, thyroid level may be checked and thyroid medicine such as Triiodothyronine may be added. Mood stabilizers including Lithium or Anticonvulsants may be used to augment. Certain Mood stabilizers require lab testing for blood levels to measure effectiveness and prevent toxicity, such as Lithium and Depakote. Others require blood draw due to side effects such as decrease in sodium level in the blood, like Carbamazepine and potentially Oxcarbazepine. Antipsychotics may be used as well. When an Antipsychotic is used, monitoring by blood draw and physical examination may be done as well due to possibility of side effects that patients may or may not be aware that they are experiencing. Some medicines have risk for increasing blood sugar and cholesterol levels. Patient may be aware of side effects such as weight gain and ExtraPyramidal Movement Symptoms, such as tremor. Please see below for commonly used augmentation medications.

Mood Stabilizers
Lithium
Anticonvulsants
Carbamazepine (Tegretol)
Gabapentin (Neurontin)
Oxcarbazepine (Trileptal)
Topiramate (Topamax)

Antipsychotics FDA Approved to Treat Depression
Aripiprazole (Abilify)
Brexpiprazole (Rexulti)
Olanzapine (Zyprexa)
Quetiapine (Seroquel XR)

Other Antipsychotics
Asenapine (Saphris)
Cariprazine (Vraylar)
Iloperidone (Fanapt)
Lurasidone (Latuda)
Paliperidone (Invega)
Risperidone (Risperdal)
Ziprasidone (Geodon)

Brain Stimulation Therapies

If you have taken at least two antidepressants for an adequate time and do not have improvement from depression, that is considered Treatment Resistant Depression. There are several FDA approved treatment options for Treatment Resistant Depression, including some of the combination options mentioned above. However, if you have tried several medicine options with little improvement, you may want to consider Brain Stimulation Therapy.

Kitty Dukakis, co-author of the book *Shock*, did not get better long term with antidepressant medicine. She required ECT, or ElectroConvulsant Therapy, in order to treat depression. ECT is a Brain Stimulation Therapy and is still a standard treatment for Treatment Resistant Depression if a patient has not improved with at least two appropriate medicines. Electrical impulses are used in ECT to create a controlled seizure in the body which allows many hormones in the brain to be released at the same time. I explain to my patients that this is like rebooting the brain, similar to rebooting a computer. Modern ECT is not like what you may have seen in the movies. The patient is prepared as if they are having a minor surgery and receive anesthesia, thus the main risk of the procedure. There is little movement of the body due to the anesthesia and muscle relaxing medicines used. Patients typically receive a series of ECT treatments in hospital before continuing treatment as an outpatient. Unfortunately, the main side effect is memory loss, particularly of events surrounding the procedure. I have actually heard of patients who have forgotten they were ever depressed.

Other Brain Stimulation Therapies FDA approved for depression include TransMagnetic Stimulation (TMS) and Vagus Nerve Stimulation (VNS). Like ECT, TMS is also thought to stimulate the brain and improve symptoms of depression. Unlike ECT, TMS uses a magnet to stimulate the brain without causing a seizure and can be done completely on an outpatient basis, for example in a physician's office. Vagus Nerve Stimulation is a medical procedure involving surgery. In VNS, an implant is placed in the chest, like a cardiac pace maker, but electrical pulses are sent to the brain by way of the vagus nerve in the neck. Patients typically experience improvement in mood over several months. A newer procedure, Magnetic Seizure Therapy is a cross between ECT and TMS. It uses a magnet to induce a seizure and has shown promising results. However, it is still in the research phase and not yet FDA approved for treatment. You may have also heard of Deep Brain Stimulation (DBS), where an implant is placed in the brain and delivers electrical pulses to help with mood. However, as of the time of this publication, DBS is not approved for depression. It is approved for relief of symptoms of Parkinson's disease and Obsessive Compulsive Disorder (OCD).

Nutrition

This section is fairly concise particularly when compared to its importance. It is listed here under medicines because the nutrients you place in your mouth go inside of your body and can cause powerful changes. According to the National Center for Complementary and Alternative Medicine (NCCAM), biologically based practices include botanicals and herbals, as well as "animal-derived extracts, vitamins, minerals, fatty acids, amino acids, proteins, prebiotics, and probiotics, whole diets, and functional foods."

The *2015 Dietary Guidelines for Americans* recommends that we eat an abundance of fresh fruits and vegetables as a part of a healthy eating pattern. Whole grains, low-fat dairy and a variety of protein are a part of this pattern of eating. Sugars, saturated fats, sodium, and alcohol should be consumed in moderation. Just as you have been tracking your mood, you can begin tracking foods you consume to see the affect nutrition has on your body. Some affects will be noticed immediately, while others take much more time. Most of us can relate to eating a large, calorie-rich meal and then feeling tired and less focused afterward. Energy rich foods can be both nutritious and flavorful, with some immediate results. However, some changes in diet and nutrition begin a series of changes at the microscopic level that may not provide noticeable affects for several months. Begin researching meal plans that provide you with nutritional facts so that you can make informed decisions about the foods you eat. If you are feeling poorly, it is likely you are eating a lot of fast food, which seems convenient and inexpensive but actually has a high cost. To purposefully plan to eat healthier is a mindset change. For example, preparing a delicious, nutritious smoothie is likely faster than ordering and receiving a delivery pizza.

Nutritional deficiencies are associated with depressive symptoms. Patients with low zinc, magnesium, folate, the B vitamins, chromium, and iron are all associated with depressive symptoms. Many of these micronutrients are needed in chemical reactions that are vital to brain growth and health. Protein intake is also important for the function of the entire body, but particularly for the brain. Amino acids are important for making proteins and several, including tryptophan, tyrosine, phenylalanine, and methionine, are thought to be helpful in treatment of depression. Two Omega-3 fatty acids, eicosapentaenoic acid (EPA) and docosahexanoic acid (DHA) have antidepressant effects. In addition to Omega-3 fatty acids, both Zinc and Magnesium, from the micronutrient list above, have been identified as being helpful in treatment of depression.

Going back to our diabetes example, a patient may check their blood sugar, determine nutritional and blood sugar milestones, and meet with a Diabetes Educator if they are having trouble with their diet. Likewise with depression, a patient should be charting mood and foods, determining their goal for symptom improvement and meet with a trained professional. While practitioners utilize a variety of approaches to treatment, some providers in particular specialize in nutritional and botanical treatments. Naturopathic providers are licensed in some states and function as primary care providers. Registered Dieticians and Nutritionists are also good sources of information about nutrition and health.

Herbs and Essential Oils

Herbal medicines can be used as an alternative to or in conjunction with conventional medicines. Remember, most of our "modern" medicine is based on the use of botanicals, such as the cardiac drug Digoxin which comes from the Digitalis (foxglove) plant. The treatment model in herbal medicine is generally different from conventional medicine. In conventional medicine, after a provider has completed a comprehensive assessment of your condition, they will give you a diagnosis and may recommend a particular medicine, likely in the form of a tablet, capsule, or caplet that has been approved by the Food and Drug Administration for a particular disease or illness. The provider will give you a prescription to take to a pharmacy, which fills the order for the medicine you will take. The Herbalist, on the other hand, will also complete a comprehensive assessment that reviews aspects of your overall wellbeing, but will not offer a diagnosis. They will listen to the concerns you have raised and provide a personalized combination of herbs, likely in the form of a tea, powder, or tincture. They then write a formula that can be compounded at a dispensary. Sometimes, depending on your preference, herbal tablets or capsules may also be used. As scientist and master's level Herbalist, Donna Koczaja states, herbs are a "subtle but powerful" treatment for certain symptoms of depression (personal communication, January 13, 2017).

One example of an herb used for depression is St. John's Wort (*Hypericum perforatum*). St. John's Wort has been studied and shown to be effective for the treatment of mild to moderate depression in certain circumstances. As with conventional medicines, it may need to be titrated to an appropriate dose. Although it is an herbal medicine, this does not mean it is not without possible interactions. In fact, St. John's Wort has been shown to interact with numerous pharmaceutical medicines including Warfarin, an anticoagulant used for treatment of blood clots in the body. Although St. John's Wort has gained popularity in recent years, consulting an Herbalist is a wise thing to do, particularly due to potential for herb-drug interactions. The herbalist monitors the latest information in the literature about product safety and is trained to check for potential interactions or allergic reactions before making recommendations. St. John's Wort is but one of many herbs that may be used to improve depression, and is not necessarily the most likely one that an herbalist will choose based on your presentation. In fact, it is likely that after they assess you, they may use an entirely different combination of medicines suited to the particular symptoms you are experiencing. As Donna Koczaja explains, the herbalist is trained to combine multiple herbs with varying actions on the body to maximize the benefit. In traditional herbal medicine, herbs are rarely employed singly.

Herbs for Depression and Stress	
Milky oats	*Avena sativa*
Skullcap	*Scutellaria laterifolia*
Holy basil/tulsi	*Ocimum sanctum*
Passionflower	*Passiflora incarnate*
Lemon Balm	*Melissa officinalis*

Essential oils are also used by practitioners to aid in health promotion. According to Violet Keys, Herbalist and Aromatherapist, essential oils can be ingested, inhaled, or absorbed through the skin, like a topical medicine (Personal communication, February 2, 2017). Essential oils are only safely ingested as aromatic herbs and spices. Prior to inhalation, it is recommended that oils be diluted. They are extremely concentrated and some can burn the skin in the case of direct contact. Topical preparations are generally provided in a diluted formulation. There is good data to support that many essential oils can help with improving mood and many other symptoms of depression. Essential oils can cause the brain to release hormones that help regulate mood. For example, inhaled sandalwood, lemon oil, and Clary sage have all been found to have some antidepressant effects.

Like other medicines, essential oils can have side effects. They are included in this section as they need to be considered in light of other substances or medicines that you intake. Many providers can now research possible interactions between medications, foods and beverages, and certain herbs.

In addition to your Psychiatrist or Mental Health provider, consider also working with a Naturopathic provider and/or Herbalist as part of your treatment team. You may need to provide signed consent for each team member to talk with each other about your care, but this is well worth the effort so that they can make informed recommendations for treatments and monitoring of blood levels as necessary for optimal health. The table below is a very brief overview of essential oils with reported uses here. Please refer to Chapter 7 for a more thorough discussion including references and source material.

Essential Oils	
Clary sage	Antidepressant effect
Lavendar	Antianxiety effect Antidepressant effect Possible pain reduction
Lavender, Lemon and Bergamot	Decrease stress Antidepressant effect Antianxiety effect
Lemon oil	Antidepressant effect Antianxiety effect
Lemon, Bergamot, Orange	Antidepressant effect
Rosemary	Possible Antidepressant effect

Questions and Answers:

Can I overcome illness without a medicine?

As was mentioned previously, some diseases are what we call "self-limited," meaning our body's immune system will fight off the illness without need of any additional medicine. Many physicians actually encourage you to allow your body to heal itself against many illnesses. If you are diagnosed with an upper respiratory infection, like the common cold, your provider may prescribe rest, fluids, and the "tincture of time." Most will not give you an antibiotic medicine because those medicines do not treat the common cold nor make the body's own process of healing occur any faster. With that said, some illnesses do require medicines to help assist our bodies in doing the work for which they were designed. If a patient chooses to treat their depression without a medicine, it is certainly possible to do so. For the best and safest result, each patient should carefully consider all of the options under the guidance of their treatment team.

How do I, as a physician, make decisions about which treatments to start with?

I try to base my initial choice on a variety of factors including patient past history of medicine use, medical history, family history, and current symptoms. For example, if a patient has family history of depression and their family member was previously helped by a particular antidepressant, I am likely recommend use of the same antidepressant. If a patient is having trouble sleeping and has a poor appetite, I might consider a Tricyclic Antidepressant, or TCA. If poor energy is a major concern, the choice of antidepressant may not be as important as a lifestyle change, such as better nutrition and a consistent exercise program.

How do I know which is the right medicine for me?

You and your provider will need to have conversations about what your symptoms are so that you can be properly diagnosed and treated. We make medical clinical decisions based on the information that we have available to us as well as the presentation that our patients give us. The combination of the history a patient provides as well as our physical examination of the patient will help your provider provide an accurate diagnosis and effective treatment plan. Other factors that are equally important are whether you can afford medicine prescribed, how the medicine is making you feel, if you have side effects, if there is a heavy pill burden, and any other concern that you have which could potentially interfere with treatment.

What do I do when I cannot seem to find the right dose or the right medicine?

If you are struggling with finding the right medicine, remember a few things. It is rare to have any medicine work completely at the initial dose. Medicines often need to be increased to effective dose to target symptoms over time. When I'm making medication changes, I try not to do more than one thing at a time. In research, we change one variable at a time, look to see the change, document and then make another change. If you're changing two or more medicines at one time, it may be unclear what is working. When you combine other non-medical interventions, use a similar approach. Try adding one thing at a time and evaluate if it is helpful. Combining a therapy with medicine is often helpful, but even this addition to treatment should be monitored for effectiveness.

How do I know if there is something more going on?

If medicine has been adjusted and you are still not getting better, you and your doctor may need to rethink your diagnosis. For example, antidepressants do not typically help long term in the context of Bipolar Disorder. Many patients can feel worse when an antidepressant is used without a mood stabilizer. If the diagnosis is correct and you have tried multiple medicines with little results, ask for genotyping, which can be done with a blood test to see if certain medicines are preferred for you. Some co-occurring illness will not get better with medicine change alone. If a person has an underlying Personality Disorder, depression may not get better, even with adequate treatment, until the Personality Disorder is treated. Intensive therapy is typically the treatment for Personality Disorders. Obviously, if a patient's condition becomes life threatening, the most urgent condition needs to be treated first.

How long should I stay on medicines?

Patients often take medications and then just stop them when they begin to feel better. Antidepressants can take four to six weeks to make changes in the cells of the brain and months to make changes to structures in the brain seen on CT and MRI. Patients often feel better within a matter of weeks and often want to quickly come off of the medicine. Because of the time it takes to create the structural brain changes even after you feel better, I typically recommend that patients continue the medications for three months from the time the begin to feel back to normal. This is most important for nutrition that is used as medicine as it also takes about three months for certain nutritional changes to take full effect in the body. The goal is for the depression to be completely treated in order to prevent recurrence of an episode of depression.

My antidepressant worked but only for a while. Now what should I do?

Most patients start out seeing a Primary Care Provider doctor who provides medicine and their depression resolves as long as they remained on the medicine long enough to prevent a recurrence. We do know that some people treated will not need to restart an antidepressant in the future. For others, the depression may recur. Some patients may need to take a higher dose of medicine, while others need to switch to a different antidepressant. Patients may need to be referred to a higher level of care if multiple medicines have been tried but with only moderate success. Consider a consultation with a provider who may have more experience with Treatment Resistant Depression, a type of depression that can be difficult to treat. Finally, there may be another underlying or co-occurring illness that needs to be further diagnosed and treated, as noted above.

What if one antidepressant is not enough?

Some patients get marked improvement with only one antidepressant. As mentioned previously, another antidepressant may be added to help deal with a symptom not managed by one medicine or to help with a side effect. Other classes of medicines can be used to augment the antidepressant, such as with a mood stabilizer or an antipsychotic. For mood stabilizers, please remember that some of these medications were originally designed to help prevent patients from having seizures. If these medicines are stopped abruptly, they could cause a seizure, even in a patient with no seizure history. Please have a conversation with your prescriber about this and other side effects that may be specific to the medicine you are using. All depression is treatable and there are other options that may be of use to you, either alone or in combination with what you are already doing.

I feel like I have tried ever medicine out there. Nothing helps. Should I give up?

Absolutely not. As mentioned before, antidepressants may not be the best treatment for everyone. As noted above, there are many options for treatment ranging from natural medicines if patients cannot or prefer not to take pills, to medical interventions such as the Brain Stimulation Therapies. You may need to be seen by a specialist, or even a sub-specialist trained in Treatment Resistant Depression. It is worth the effort. Depression is a treatable illness and you can get better.

My doctor added a medicine to my antidepressant. What do I need to know about this new medicine?

Your provider wants to help you get better. They may add a medicine to help boost the effect of antidepressants in some patients. They are not antidepressants themselves, but have been shown in some cases to help patients on an antidepressant feel better than when on an antidepressant alone. Antipsychotic medications are fairly popular now due to direct-to-consumer advertising. Sometimes called Atypical Antipsychotics, and otherwise known as Second Generation Antipsychotics, these medicines were designed to help people with symptoms of psychosis. If in the context of your depression you also see or hear things others do not see and hear, or feel very paranoid and fearful for no explainable reason, a provider may add an Antipsychotic medication for a period of time. There is a risk of Movement Disorders, such as tremor and internal feeling of restlessness, as well as possible weight gain with certain medicines, so again, discuss the risk and benefit with your provider. If you have an underlying medical condition such as Diabetes or High Cholesterol, there is risk of worsening these conditions. There is a risk of worsening blood sugar or having blood cholesterol increased. For that reason, it is recommended to check glucose, or sugar levels, cholesterol levels, and in some cases liver and kidney function if you have some underlying medical conditions.

My medicine doesn't seem to be helping with all of my depression symptoms. What do I do?

Expect that a medicine will help lift your mood and improve your outlook on life. Some symptoms of depression resolve quicker than others. Typically I share that within the first week, irritability decreases, followed by mood improvement in the next several weeks. Over time, sleep, appetite, energy and concentration will also improve. Some symptoms can linger longer than others. Charting your moods will help you see when certain symptoms improve and also determine if other systems need to be in place to address symptoms that medicines do not. Remember medications alone may not address every symptom of depression. I wish I had an easy answer for problems with motivation, procrastination, etc. Other systems have to be in place to address things like procrastination and motivation, unless these strictly occurred only as a part of the depression. As mentioned above and discussed more thoroughly in Chapter 7, some essential oils may help with symptoms that may occur along with depression.

I have an Anxiety Disorder, but my doctor prescribed an Antidepressant. Why is that?

Depression and Anxiety typically occur along the same spectrum. Treatment with an antidepressant helps with depression, but is also used in Anxiety Disorders. The dose usually does need to be higher to help with anxiety. As noted earlier, some treatments thought to potentially help with depression are actually approved for Anxiety Disorders.

CHAPTER 5

Staying Better Longer:

Pursuing Peace with the Self and Others

"It isn't enough to talk about peace. One must believe in it. And it isn't enough to believe in it. One must work at it."

– Eleanor Roosevelt

I want to congratulate you again for sticking with the process of getting and staying better. Dealing with depression is not typically a fun topic. Be mindful of the fact that depression can reoccur in some cases and guarding against it is well worth your time and energy. The focus of this chapter is on leaving a trail of "bread crumbs" for you to follow in the future should symptoms attempt to return. In the latter portion of the chapter, making peace with the past in a healthy way is also discussed.

As you move away from the grip of depression, you may be fearful of symptoms returning. This is where I want you to focus on leaving those breadcrumbs and pebbles for yourself. In the story of *Hansel and Gretel*, the brother and sister wander from home, but leave a trail behind so that they can find their way back. As the story is told, at one point they leave breadcrumbs that are eaten by birds so they have difficulty finding their way home and become lost in the dark woods. However, when they leave white pebbles, they more easily find their way back.

In most countries, bread is a staple for life. Though temporary, it helps sustain life for the time that it is available to be consumed. There are coping methods that you have used, and although they provided temporary satisfaction, they helped lift the veil of depression long enough to provide hope to make it to another day. I honor whatever you have done to bring you to the place that you are today. You did not quit on life, and life has not quit on you. For the Christian, recall the words of Christ who said "I am the bread of life." (John Chapter 6:35) Meditate on this as one type of bread that does provide a permanent trail to be followed.

The pebbles from the *Hansel and Gretel* story are an example of a more permanent source back to health. These tangible reminders were helpful and not as easily removed by external factors. Have there been things you have used that provided temporary relief, but were unhealthy? Instead of leaving pebbles for yourself, you have used breadcrumbs and lost your way. If so, make a decision to replace those unhealthy coping methods with healthier behaviors discussed in Chapters 3 and 4. Much of your system may still be of use. No experience is wasted experience. Write down methods that have helped you previously, but really focus on the things you want to keep as pebbles to return to again and again.

Once healthy methods are written down, place them in a prominent place that can be seen often as a helpful reminder. Incorporate the methods it into your system. Set up reminders and leave them for yourself. For example, keeping a prominent picture readily in view, having a recurring event on your phone calendar, or putting things in a mini-time capsule can all be effective ways of leaving reminders for you. These things are a gift to yourself for a future time when you are faced with negative thoughts that try to lead you back to depression. Your system that you develop will not only help you get better faster, but also help you stay better longer.

Gaining and keeping the victory you have obtained thus far does not mean you will not have challenges ahead. Processing some of the factors involved in becoming depressed is important. One associated factor some patients experience is anger, in the form of irritability. While not all patients experience this, several pioneering Psychiatrists including Dr. Sigmund Freud have expressed that depression is anger turned inward. For patients who do experience significant anger at themselves or others, defining where the anger is coming from is a necessary step towards wholeness. Let's return to the analogy about my patients who have been incarcerated. Most struggle with anger and have a hard time letting go of it. If we process feelings associated with anger, we often find hurt and unfairness as common themes.

When we trace it back to the place when they were first hurt, or disrespected, it is not long before a history of negative events unfolds, such as abuse or trauma. Often, they have been taken advantage of when they were too vulnerable to ward against it, and now have determined that they will not be hurt or disrespected again. If they could go back in the past and deal with the original person or issue that caused them the harm, they would well be on their way to overcoming the anger, and likely the depression.

This is where we begin to talk about forgiveness. People share that they have a hard time letting go of the person or event that caused emotional or physical hurt. Why is forgiveness important? Let me share a quote with you about the results of a lack of forgiveness and its relationship to anger.

"Of the Seven Deadly Sins, anger is possibly the most fun. To lick your wounds, to smack your lips over grievances long past, to roll over your tongue the prospect of bitter confrontations still to come, to savor to the last toothsome morsel both the pain you are given and the pain you are giving back -- in many ways it is a feast fit for a king. The chief drawback is that what you are wolfing down is yourself. The skeleton at the feast is you."

- Frederick Buechner

Holding onto the hurt and anger from the harm others have done to you actually leaves you drowning in bitterness. It continually reopens wounds so that they cannot heal properly. Before we address how to go about the process of healing, let me remind you of what forgiveness is not. It is not excusing a person from the harm they have done. It is not a feeling, rather it is an action. It is relinquishing your right to punish an offender for what they have done. In the treatment of depression, particularly that related to loss or trauma, I will work with a person on the process of "letting go" of this particular right, and reaching forward to their next stage of growth.

This is why I call this process "forward giving." The gift of forgiveness is something you give to yourself. Making peace with your past, and those that have wronged you gives you the freedom to move forward with your life unhindered by your past. Being unburdened by past hurts allows you to pursue peace with others and just as importantly, peace with yourself.

Some wonder about how to address the person who has offended them. In cases other than trauma and abuse, it is recommended that the process begin fairly quickly so that a small emotional wound is not allowed to fester into a larger more complicated wound. When abuse or trauma has occurred, confronting a perpetrator takes thoughtfulness and preparation. I counsel patients against this until we carefully consider both the patient's expected response as well as the offender's response. I have found in some cases, confrontation does more harm than good, particularly if my patient is in a fragile or vulnerable place mentally. Sometimes circumstances, such as death or incarceration hinder confronting a perpetrator, but it does not need to hinder the forgiveness process. Forgiveness can still occur. Whatever you decide, work with a trusted therapist or support person, preferably one trained or experienced in trauma recovery.

When patients are in treatment with me for trauma-related events, it is recommended they write a letter to the person that has offended or wronged them first. The letter is reviewed with myself or a trusted person. We then discuss whether or not the letter needs to be sent. For some, just the process of working through the emotions they put on paper is enough. The letter can then be ceremoniously burned, torn, or buried. For others, the letter can be sent, but we discuss the implications of a response versus no response at all. We review the letter for safety, both for the patient and the perpetrator. While my patient is my concern, we do not want to send anything that could be considered a threat to a perpetrator. After this process, patients usually feel as if they have gone through a cleansing, or a catharsis. They have shared that the process is quite helpful for them.

Visualization may help with this. In your mind, imagine having a fishing pole with line and fish hook at the end. Imagine the offensive event that has happened to you as a fishing lure. Put it on the fishing hook, and cast it into the sea of forgetfulness. This is not to say you throw all the helpful lessons learned into the sea, just the event that attempted to scar you beyond recognition.

Do not be discouraged when you have forgiven for something and it appears to rear its head again, as if you did not do a good enough job the first time. Forgiveness is a process. If a stranger on the street bumps into you and asks forgiveness, you will likely give it and move on your way without giving the incident another thought. However, if an intimate person you trusted has betrayed you, that is a different story. You may now need to go through the process of forgiving the person for hurting you, for dishonoring the intimacy that had been developed, for betraying your trust, and for the event that occurred. As you grow and mature in character, you may find the need to offer forgiveness again based on the growth you have experienced. Please consider taking at least a step of forgiveness as it releases you from being the skeleton at the feast of anger and depression.

CHAPTER 6

Healing

"There is a light in this world, a healing spirit more powerful than any darkness we may encounter"

– Mother Teresa

The story is told of a man who needed surgery to repair a badly injured knee. The man asked the surgeon "how long would it take the knee to be completely healed after the surgery?" The surgeon replied, "I will do the surgery, but it's up to God to do the healing." I think that was a wise response. There is a limit to modern medicine. Providers do the very best we can by our patients, but we do not have all of the answers. I believe that where we end in our abilities, that is where God, or your Higher Power, begins.

There are many laws, or principles, we borrow from the Bible and use for our benefit, Christian or not. Apparently after Shakespeare, the Bible is the most commonly quoted source material in English. You have heard of phrases like "a broken heart," "a labor of love," a drop in the bucket," "by the skin of my teeth," and getting to "the root of the matter." These phrases all originated in the King James Version of the Bible. In terms of lessons we can use for life, many have heard in some form or another, the teaching about the wise ant that works hard during the summer to store up food for the winter. Well, this teaching was written by the wisest and wealthiest man in the world, King Solomon, in his writings collectively known as Proverbs.

There are a host of scriptures on healing of illnesses recorded in the Bible, including wise sayings about depression. Dodie Osteen, mother of current Pastor Joel Osteen, lists scriptures focused on healing that were of benefit to her in her book *Healed of Cancer*. Several scriptures and positive affirmations are included below. If you are unfamiliar with the Bible, the first name listed is the name of the book. The number followed by the colon is the chapter followed by the verse. If you do not feel comfortable with scriptures, focus on the positive quotes or affirmations. However, please remember that these scriptures make no distinction between a Christian and a non-Christian and benefits can be for both. How is this possible? Well, consider thinking about it this way. The Bible is the single oldest surviving document to have both characters and geographic locations contained in its text confirmed by multiple outside historical texts of its time. Truths that are found within its pages are in parallel not only to other cultures and faith belief systems, but have information that can be of benefit to all. If you are of the Jewish faith, you may not feel comfortable using the New Testament, and prefer the Torah. You may want to focus on only Old Testament scriptures as these are based on the Torah. If you are atheist or agnostic, you may feel more comfortable focusing less on scriptural materials, and more on the positive quotes. Use this material to help build your armament of positive affirmations that you position in prominent places to focus, meditate on, and eventually memorize. Find a way to make them your own. Then when difficult times come, it will have less effect on your mindset and your mood.

As you read below, remember that the Bible comes in different versions, or translations, of the original language. The overall meaning from one version to another is the same when translated in context. My language of origin and comfort is English, but I appreciate the beauty of the French language or stateliness of the Russian language. The King James Version (KJV) is written in Old English and has certain poetry to it. So as not to be lost in translation, the Amplified (AMP) lists many of the meanings of Hebrew or Greek words in parenthesis that cannot be simply translated as one word in English. Both the Message (MSG) and New International Version (NIV) use more modern English and many find this easier to understand and relate. The scriptures below are listed in one of these four versions, or languages.

As believers we know that the Bible promises healing of all sickness, illness, and disease. We are told to ask in prayer for healing and then give thanksgiving in faith for what we asked (1 Thessalonians Chapter 5:18). King David did this often. He began many songs, or Psalms, with an honest account of his feelings, but then he seems to abruptly turn the focus from himself to his God, offering praise for things that God had already done and for the future things he had faith that He would do. Many have noticed benefit from turning their hurting hearts towards helping others. Again, this takes the focus off of you, ultimately helping with your healing process and that of others. For some, you will experience healing swiftly. For others, the process may take longer and a medicine or other intervention is helpful. Recall the surgeon's example above. I do not know why for some people in biblical times only a spoken word or a touch was needed, while for others a "balm" and further "faith in action" was needed. Just as the wise surgeon had to admit his limitations in knowing when healing would take place, I have to concede that I also have limitations in knowing when it will occur for my patients. What I do know is that healing is possible.

"The greatest healing therapy is friendship and love." Hubert Humphrey

"A happy heart is good medicine and a joyful mind causes healing, But a broken spirit dries up the bones" Proverbs 17: 22 (AMP)

"Healing comes when we choose to walk away from darkness and move towards a brighter light." – Dieter Uchtdorf

"Light in a messenger's eyes brings joy to the heart, and good news gives health to the bones" Proverbs 15: 20 (NIV)

"The happiness of your life depends upon the quality of your thoughts; therefore guard accordingly." – Marcus Aurelius

"My son, attend to my words; consent and submit to my sayings. Let them no depart from your sight; keep them in the center of your heart, for they are life to those who find them, healing and health to all their flesh" Proverbs 4: 20 - 22 (AMP)

"In the midst of difficulty lies opportunity." - Albert Einstein

"As Jesus entered the village of Capernaum, a Roman captain came up in a panic and said, "Master, my servant is sick. He cannot walk. He's in terrible pain." Jesus said, "I will come and heal him." "Oh, no," said the captain. "I don't want to put you to all that trouble. Just give the order and my servant will be fine. I'm a man who takes orders and gives orders. I tell one soldier, 'Go,' and he goes; to another,' Come," and he comes; to my slave, 'Do this,' and he does it." The Jesus turned to the captain and said, "Go. What you believed could happen has happened." At that moment his servant became well." Matthew 8: 5 - 9, 13. (MSG)

"Tell your heart that the fear of suffering is worse than suffering itself. And no heart has ever suffered when it goes in search of its dream." – Paulo Coelho

"I am holding you by your right, I, the Lord your God. I say to you, Do not be afraid. I am here to help you." Isaiah 41: 13 (AMP)

"Although the world is full of suffering, it is also full of the overcoming of it." – Helen Keller

"You have kept track of my every toss and turn through the sleepless nights, each tear entered in your ledger, each ache written in your book. God, you did everything you promised, and I'm thanking you with all my heart. You pulled me from the brink of death, my feet from the cliff-edge of doom. Now I stroll at leisure with God in the sunlit fields of life" Psalm 56: 8, 12 -13 (MSG)

"Every positive thought propels you in the right direction." – Elizabeth Kipp

"Have mercy on me and be gracious to me, O Lord, for I am weak (faint, frail); Heal me, O Lord, for my bones are dismayed and anguished" Psalm 6:2 (AMP)

"The words of kindness are more healing to a drooping heart than balm or honey." – Sarah Fielding

Heal me, O Lord, and I will be healed. Save me and I will be saved. For You are my praise" Jeremiah 17: 14 (AMP)

"There is no key to happiness. The door is always open." – Mother Teresa

"Then He touched their eyes, saying, "According to your faith [your trust and confidence in My power and My ability to heal] it will be done to you" Matthew 9: 29 (AMP)

"Hope is the thing with feathers that perches in the soul and sings the tune without the words and never stops at all." –Emily Dickinson

"I create the fruit of the lips. Peace, peace to him that is far off, and to him that is near, saith the Lord, and I will heal him" Isaiah 57: 19 (KJV)

"If you are willing to do only what is easy, life will be hard, but if you are willing to do what's hard, life will be easy." T. Harv Eker

"He sends forth His word and heals them and rescues them from the pit and destruction" Psalm 107: 20 (AMP)

"Only in the darkness can you see the stars." - Martin Luther King, Jr

"God is our refuge and strength, a very present help in trouble" Psalm 46: 1 (KJV)

"Affliction brings out graces that cannot be seen in a time of health. It is the treading of the grapes that brings out the sweet juices of the vine." – Robert Murray McCheyne

"Whither shall I go from thy spirit? Or whither shall I flee from thy presence? If I ascend up into heaven, thou are there; if I make my bed in hell, behold, thou art there. If I take the wings of the morning, and dwell in the uttermost parts of the sea; even there shall thy hand lead me, and thy right hand shall hold me" Psalms 139: 7 - 10 (KJV)

"Without a struggle, there can be no progress."- Frederick Douglass

"Do not fear [anything], for I am with you; do not be afraid, for I am your God. I will strengthen you, be assured I will help you. I will certainly take hold of you with My righteous right hand [a hand of justice, of power, of victory, of salvation]" Isaiah 41: 10 (AMP)

"If you are going through hell, keep going." – Winston Churchill

"Surely He has borne our griefs (sicknesses, weaknesses, and distresses) and carried our sorrows and pains (of punishment)...He was wounded for our transgression, He was bruised for our guilt and iniquities; the chastisement [needful to obtain] our peace was upon Him and with the stripes [that wounded] Him we are healed and made whole" Isaiah 53: 4 - 5 (AMP)

"For every minute you remain angry, you give up sixty seconds of peace of mind." - Ralph Waldo Emerson

"Who forgives all of your iniquities, who heals all your diseases?" Psalm 103:3

"In three words I can sum up everything I have learned about life: it goes on." - Robert Frost

"For I will restore health to you, and I will heal your wounds, says the Lord" Jeremiah 30:17a (AMP)

"I used to believe that prayer changes things, but now I know that prayer changes us, and we change things." - Mother Teresa

"Now Jesus called together the twelve [disciples] and gave them [the right to exercise] power and authority over all the demons and to heal diseases" Luke 9: 1 (AMP)

"Healing is a matter of time, but it is sometimes also a matter of opportunity." - Hippocrates

"The Spirit of the God, the Master, is on me because God anointed me. He sent me to preach good news to the poor, heal the brokenhearted, announce freedom to all captives, and pardon all prisoners" Isaiah 61: 1 - 2 (MSG)

"There is no exercise better for the heart than reaching down and lifting people up." – John Andrew Holmes, Jr

"The Spirit of the Lord is upon me, because he hath anointed me to preach the gospel to the poor; he hath sent me to heal the brokenhearted, to preach deliverance to the captives and recovering of sight to the blind, to set at liberty them that are bruised, to preach the acceptable year of the Lord" Luke 4:18 - 19 (KJV)

"I prayed for twenty years but received no answer until I prayed with my legs." -Frederick Douglass

"Thou will keep him in perfect peace, whose mind is stayed on thee because he trusted in Thee" Isaiah 26: 3 (KJV)

"Optimism is the faith that leads to achievement. Nothing can be done without hope and confidence." - Helen Keller

"I shall not die but live, and shall declare the works and recount the illustrious acts of the Lord" Psalm 118: 7 (AMP)

"Broken crayons still color." – Author Unknown

"With long life will I satisfy him and show him My salvation" Psalm 91: 16 (AMP)

"...and your very flesh shall be a great poem." – Walt Whitman

"And a leper came up to Him and bowed down before Him, saying "Lord, if You are willing, You are able to make me clean (well)." Jesus reached out His hand and touched him, saying, "I am willing; be cleansed." Immediately, his leprosy was cleansed" Matthew 8: 2 - 3 (AMP)

"There is more wisdom in your body than in your deepest philosophies." –Friedrich Nietzsche

"For God did not give us a spirit of timidity or cowardice or fear; but [He has given us a spirit] of power and of love and of sound judgment and personal discipline [abilities that result in a calm, well-balanced mind and self-control]" 2 Timothy 1: 7 (AMP)

"Your success and happiness lies in you. Resolve to keep happy, and your joy and you shall form an invincible host against difficulties." - Helen Keller

CHAPTER 7

The Art and Science

"Principles for the Development of a Complete Mind: Study the science of art. Study the art of science. Develop your senses – especially learn how to see. Realize that everything connects to everything else."

-Leonardo da Vinci

You may have noticed that the initial chapters were lighter reading compared to the latter chapters. If you are like me, when you are not feeling your best, you have little to no desire to read an exhaustive text. You want the answer to your question, or at least a push in the right direction to find your answer as quickly and efficiently as possible. However, if you are inquisitive like I am, you also want to know "the reason behind the reason" as I once heard a consultant say. Once I am feeling better, I will read further to find out why things work the way they do. If it's a drug, what is its mechanism of action? If it's an essential oil, what part of the brain is it supposed to work in and why? To be as clear as possible, I gave information in proceeding chapters on what I have found to work for patients, and for myself, without weighting the text down with references or too much explanation as to the studies behind what works.

In this chapter, I repeat information from our scaffold but add many more details as it relates to building on what you already know. This is not to be redundant, but to give more insight into the studies behind information already presented so that you know what I have shared up to this point is true, at least at the time this edition is published. Yes, science continues to advance, and we continue to make new and exciting discoveries every single day. This is a good thing. Do not be discouraged if you see or hear of reference to a study that shows one result today and two years from now another shows a different result. The studies may be looking at things from different angles, or our knowledge base will have expanded. Take the information in stride - it is growing, just like you. You will notice sentences may end in parentheses with the name of an author of the study as well as the year published (i.e. Scientist, 2016).

This chapter concludes with references and at the conclusion of the book is a resource section alluded to in previous chapters. Please note that as we discussed before, education and moderation is the key. Now that you are feeling better, take time to research organizations or groups before joining. If you do decide to join or follow a group, use moderation. It is better to join one group that you commit to checking into daily or weekly, than following ten groups that send you notifications constantly and you get nothing done because you get bombarded and distracted by too many messages Yes, I have been there and it is not helpful for most people.

In the science of medicine, we move from having an idea, or hypothesis, and testing this initially in a lab or under a controlled setting to replicating the results of the study. If we have found the results to be helpful, we then move to what is known as translational research, or moving from seeing if something works in a laboratory to seeing if it works among select patients and eventually an entire population by virtue of clinical trial. This process can easily take years to complete in a safe manner. Any antidepressant that is approved by the Food and Drug Administration (FDA) has gone through this process and been shown to significantly reduce depression when compared to placebo, or what some people used to call a sugar pill. Each clinical study, sometimes several for the same drug, must be critically reviewed for understanding. However, this is just the beginning.

There is a term in laboratory medicine called "too numerous to count," meaning that the number of cells being counted are beyond what can be detected and individuated by the human eye or by use of a computer. The same is true of the myriad of articles available related to effectiveness of antidepressant medicines. Anti-depressant medicines, Electro Convulsive Therapy (ECT), Vagus Nerve Stimulation (VNS) and Trans Magnetic Stimulation (TMS) are all FDA approved for treatment of depression and have been shown to be effective in multiple studies. For that reason, the references below are predominantly for lesser known and non-conventional medical treatments. This is to stimulate conversation between you and your provider. If you have questions about success in the scientific literature about a particular medicine, please discuss this with your provider.

An antidepressant in combination with therapy continues to have the greatest benefit for many (Schwartz, 2016). While the neurotransmitter serotonin is thought to be low in depression and increased with most antidepressants, other neurotransmitters such as dopamine and norepinephrine are also beneficial. Serotonin is thought to be a large contributor to feelings of well-being and happiness, and its dietary precursor is the amino acid Tryptophan (Lv, 2013). Serotonin can also be increased using exercise and mental techniques (Siqueira, 2016, Korb, 2011).

Reflecting on past positive accomplishments has been shown to increase this hormone. Exposure to sunlight increases both Serotonin and Vitamin D. Serotonin's precursor Tryptophan is an amino acid found in the diet that can cross the blood brain barrier, a barrier between the body's blood system and the brain. Dopamine is one of the pleasure hormones, increasing when your needs and desires are met (Breuning, 2012). Visualization of a goal and then accomplishing it, no matter how small, will help release this hormone. St John's Wort appears to inhibit reuptake of serotonin, dopamine, and norepinephrine thereby increasing these neurotransmitters' availability in the brain, similar to antidepressants (Jorm, 2002).

Endorphins, released during stress and pain, help block pain and can also be increased with exercise (Zschuck, 2013). Other fun activities that increase Endorphins include eating dark chocolate, laughter, and the essential oils vanilla and lavender (see below). Oxytocin is involved with social interactions, including bonding and development of trust. It is helpful in facial recognition of emotions, and activities such as spending intimate time with another can increase oxytocin. Interaction with others does not necessarily mean human. Time spent with pets and plants can be just as rewarding. Currently, research is underway that indicates intranasal oxytocin may be an effective treatment for depression (Hofmann, 2015). S-

Adenosylmethionine (SAMe) is an amino acid derivative that has been shown in at least one study to have similar effects to the tricyclic antidepressant Imipramine. It has been approved for use in Australia (Jorm, 2002).

These hormones do not work alone in the body, but rather go to structures in the brain, most notably the limbic system. The Limbic system includes structures such as the hippocampus, amygdala, and hypothalamus. The hippocampus is the memory center, the amygdala is the "seat of the emotions," and the hypothalamus links hormones to the nervous system. The hippocampus has been shown to decrease in size in patient with depression. Creation of new cells, or neurogenesis, in our hippocampus, is increased under treatment with antidepressants. Brain-derived neurotrophic factor (BDNF) may be involved (Liu, 2015). In both geographic location and function, these structures are near to the olfactory bulb, which detects smell and the nucleus accumbens, the pleasure center of the brain.

The olfactory bulb is a structure that can change based on sensory input. In Negoias' 2010 paper, among German hospitalized patients diagnosed with major depressive disorder, mostly women and mostly on psychotropic medication, they were found to have smaller olfactory bulb volumes and this correlated with depression scores from the Beck Depression Inventory (Negoias, 2010). Meaning, there may be a potential olfactory deficit, or decreased sense of smell in patients with clinical depression. Reduced sense of smell has been connected to abnormal disinhibition, or difficulties turning off, the amygdala, which is the emotional center of the brain responsible for learning and modulating emotions, such as sadness and fear (Pause, 2001). It is unclear if patients with depression develop the olfactory deficit, or if olfactory deficits predispose such patients to developing depression. What the German study did show is that after depression was treated, patient's olfactory response was not statistically different from the non-depressed patients.

In Boldrini's 2009 paper based on autopsy results, patients with major depressive disorder treated with either SSRIs or TCAs in the last three months of life based on toxicology, or level of drug in the system, were compared to those with major depressive disorder without medications, or drug detected in the system (Boldrini, 2009). Those treated with antidepressants, regardless of category, had increased neuron precursor cells, and larger volume of the area of the hippocampus studied.

Multiple antidepressants of different classes have been shown to enhance adult hippocampal neurogenesis; According to a UK study, sertraline seems to do so by a glucocorticoid receptor (Anackler, 2011). This receptor action begins a cascade that affects the nucleus of the cell, the DNA contained inside, and ultimately, transcription of genetic material thought to help in ultimate treatment of depression. Exercise, environmental enrichment, and learning increase neurogenesis, or neuron development in the hippocampus.

We discussed the National Center for Complementary and Alternative Medicine (NCCAM) guideline in Chapter 4. For completeness, NCCAM definition of Mind-Body Medicine includes "the interactions among the brain, mind, body, and behavior, and the powerful ways in which emotional, mental, social, spiritual, and behavioral factors can directly affect health." It includes some interventions previously discussed but more commonly thought of as psychological techniques or therapies, such as relaxation, visual imagery, and Cognitive Behavioral Therapies.

Whole medicine systems are "complete systems of theory and practice that developed independently" from conventional modern medicine, but may still be used in parallel (Guidance for Industry, 2016). While the Dietary Supplement Health and Education Act of 1994 (DSHEA) is legislature that regulates the manufacturing of dietary supplements and herbals, licensure of practitioners is not mandated in all states and for all medicine systems. The legal definition of dietary supplement according to DSHEA includes "vitamins, minerals, herbs or other botanicals, amino acids, and substances such as enzymes, organ tissues, glandulars, and metabolites. Dietary supplements can also be extracts or concentrates, and may be found in many forms such as tablets, capsules, softgels, gelcaps, liquids, or powders."

It is well known that Thyroid conditions can mimic and co-occur in depression. Nutrient deficiency can also mimic depression. Both low Zinc and Magnesium have been associated with depression and when they are replenished, depression symptoms decrease (Greenblatt, 2016). As noted above SAMe is helpful for treatment of depression. Omega 3 fatty acids, eicosapentaenoic acid (EPA) and docosahexenoic acid (DHA), are thought to be helpful in the treatment of depression (Evans, 2016). The Omega 3 alpha-linolenic acid, contained in nuts and plant oils, gets converted to EPA and DHA, which are thought to work as anti-inflammatory agents. EPA and DHA can be obtained from eating cold-water fish.

Vitamins and supplements have become increasingly popular for both health maintenance and the treatment of depression. Tryptophan is a precursor to serotonin, and methionine is a precursor to S-adenosylmethionine, or SAMe. S-adenosylmethionine (SAMe) is an amino acid derivative that has been shown in at least one study to have similar effects to the Tricyclic Antidepressant Imipramine. It has been approved for use in Australia (Jorm, 2002). Omega-3 may help in reducing inflammation, as systemic inflammation has been associated with several symptoms of depression including low energy, loss of interest, poor appetite, and sleep disturbance (Evans, 2017). Zinc has been found to be low in patients with depression, and augmentation of zinc with antidepressant therapy has been shown to improve symptoms of depression (Greenblatt, 2017). Magnesium helps modify your body's response to stress, and has been found to be helpful both as adjunctive treatment and as monotherapy when compared to the antidepressant Imipramine.

Knowing the importance of the relationship between smell, olfactory bulb function, and Hippocampal cells, this may explain why use of essential oils may be helpful in depression and other illnesses. In a 2013 article, researchers at Xiamen University in China made the observation below in their abstract:

"Most studies, as well as clinically applied experience, have indicated that various essential oils, such as lavender, lemon and bergamot can help to relieve stress, anxiety, depression and other mood disorders. Most notably, inhalation of essential oils can communicate signals to the olfactory system and stimulate the brain to exert

neurotransmitters (e.g. serotonin and dopamine) thereby further regulating mood." (Lv, 2013).

Researchers have found that a mixture of Bergamot, Orange and Lemon (with Lemon predominating) that was slowly vaporized throughout the day over a two-week period helped patient with Depression reduce their dose of antidepressants (Komori, 1995). In a separate study of hospice patients, humidified lavender resulted in patient's reporting reduced subjective rating of depression, anxiety, and pain, and improved overall sense of well-being (Lewis, 2002). Additionally, these patients had some lowering of blood pressure and pulse. The results, based on one hour long treatment, were not statistically significant, but the trend appeared promising. Of note, lavender appears to have more success with Anxiety co-occurring with Depression as opposed to benefit for treatment of Depression alone.

Lemon oil is thought to decrease levels of the stress hormones, and have antidepressant affects, possibly by increasing turnover of serotonin (Lv, 2013, Dobetsberger, 2011). In a 2014 study published in the Journal of Phytotherapy, inhalation of Clary Sage resulted in decreased cortisol levels, and increased serotonin, and improved thyroid function. The Korean study was conducted with post-menopausal women and was thought to have significant effect on depression showing improved mood as measured by the Korean version of the Beck Depression Inventory (Lee, 2014). Rosemary oil has been found to act on serotonin receptors (Martinez et al 2009).

Any product applied to the skin should be used with caution. They can still interact with the other medicines that you take internally. In addition to inhaling essential oils, some patients participate in use of oils as aromatherapy with massage. Remember than in either case, oils are often diluted prior to use. There is mixed support of massage alone versus addition of aromatherapy to achieve better results. For completeness, consider the 2016 Cochrane review of use of massage with and without aromatherapy among patients with cancer. These reviews were conducted with multiple different types of fragrances of oils. The review concluded that based on the limited data available to then, they were unable to assess an added benefit of aromatherapy versus massage alone (Shin, 2016).

Some practitioners that use supplements noted above also have limited prescribing privileges compared to those trained in conventional medicine. For example, Naturopathic providers function similar to a Primary Care Physician, such as in the state of Vermont. Herbalists are also providers of care that use botanicals as well. Though there is currently no state licensing available, these providers are trained in the use of herbs. Some practitioners study traditional homeopathy, a particular branch of treatments, but the World Health Organization warned against its use for treating serious diseases related to limited scientific data demonstrating health benefits (Mashta, 2009, Ernst, 2002). Please see the Resource section for more information about organizations that provide information about and for Naturopathic providers or Herbalists.

Regardless of the type of medicine that you use, it should be discussed with your care provider and utilized as recommended for the most effective outcome. We have discussed many tools that you can use to help you along your journey. While not everything that we have discussed will uniquely fit you, it is my hope that you have gained useful information that has helped you achieve success, especially as it relates to overcoming depression. You have now made it to the completion of this comparatively brief book on ways to have victory over depression. In the section following this chapter, please find a list of resources, including organizations that will help you maintain what you have accomplished.

Scientific References

2008 Physical Activity Guidelines for Americans. US Department of Health and Human Services https://health.gov/paguidelines/guidelines/ October 2008 Accessed January 24, 2017.

Akhondzadeh Basti A, Moshiri E, Noorbala AA, et al (2007). Comparison of petal of Crocus sativus L. and fluoxetine in the treatment of depressed outpatients: a pilot double-blind randomized trial. Prog Neuropsychopharmacol Biol Psychiatry. 31:439-42.

Anackler, C, Zunszain, P, Cattaneo, A, Carvalho, A, et al (2011). Antidepressants Increase Human Hippocampal Neurogenesis by Activating the Glucocorticoid Receptor. Molecular Psychiatry 16, 738-750.

Boldrini M, Underwood MD, Hen R, Rosoklija GB, et al (2009). Antidepressants Increase Neural Progenitor Cells in the Human Hippocampus. Neuropsychopharmacology 34(11):2376 –2389.

Breuning, L. (Posted December 8, 2012) Five Ways to Boost Your Natural Happy Chemicals. Psychology Today.

Buschhuter D, Smitka M, Dobetsberger, C and Buchbauer, G. (2011) Actions of Essential Oils on the Central Nervous System: An Updated Review. Flavor and Fragrance Journal 26:300-316

Dobetsberger, C and Buchbauer, G. (2011) Actions of Essential Oils on the Central Nervous System: An Updated Review. Flavor and Fragrance Journal. 26:300-316

Ernst E. (2002) A systematic review of systematic reviews of homeopathy. Br J Clin Pharmacol. Dec;54(6):577-82.

Evans, S, Edwards, L. (2016) Fat, Food, and Mood: Beyond Omega-3s. Psychiatric Times. December: 17-19.

Greenblatt, J, To, W, Dimino, J. (2016) Evidenced-Based Research on the Role of Zinc and Magnesium Deficiencies in Depression. Psychiatric Times. December: 11-13.

Guidance for Industry: Complementary and Alternative Medicine Products and Their Regulation by the Food and Drug Administration (2016) US Department of Health and Human Services. Food and Drug Administration. December 2016. Draft document: pages 2-3, 6. Accessed January 21, 2017.

Hofmann, SG, Fang, A Brager, D. (2015) Effect of Intranasal Oxytocin Administration on Psychiatric Symptoms: A Meta-analysis of Placebo-controlled Studies. Psychiatry Reserch. August; 228(3):708-14.

Jorm, A, Christensen, H, Griffiths, K, Rodgers, B. (2002) Effectiveness of Complementary and Self-help Treatments for Depression. Medical Journal of Australia 176 (10): 84.

Korb, Alex. (2011) Boosting Your Serotonin Activity: Four Ways to Boost your Serotonin. Psychology Today. (Posted November 17, 2011. Accessed January 6, 2017.

Komori T, Fujiwara R, Tanida M, Nomura J. (1995) Potential antidepressant effects of lemon odor in rats. Eur Neuropsychopharmacol. Dec;5(4):477-80.

Kowatch, R, Monroe, E, Delgado, S. (2011) Not All Mood Swings are Bipolar Disorder. Current Psychiatry. February 2011 10(2): 38-B

Lee, K, Cho, E, Kang, Y. (2014) Changes in 5-Hydroxytryptamine and Cortisol Plasma Levels in Menopausal Women after Inhalation of Clary Sage Oil. Physiotherapy Research 28:1599-1605.

Lewis, M and Kowalski, S. (December 2002) American Journal of Hospice & Palliative Care 19(6): 381-386.

132

Liu, L, Liu, C, Wang, Y, Wang, Pu, (2015) Herbal Medicine for Anxiety, Depression and Insomnia. Current Neuropharmacology July 13(4): 481–493.

Lv, X, Liu, Z, Zhang, H, Tzeng, CM. (2013) Aromatherapy and the Central Nerve System (CNS): Therapeutic Mechanism and Its Associated Genes. Current Drug Targets 14(8):872-879.

Martínez AL, González-Trujano ME, Pellicer F, López-Muñoz FJ, Navarrete A. (2009) Antinociceptive effect and GC/MS analysis of Rosmarinus officinalis L. essential oil from its aerial parts. Planta Med. Apr;75(5):508-11.

Mashta O. (2009) WHO warns against using homoeopathy to treat serious diseases. BMJ. Aug 24;339:b3447.

Negoias S, Croy I, Gerber J, Puschmann, Petroweski K, Joraschky P, Hummel T. (2010)

Reduced Olfactory Bulb Volume and Olfactory Sensitivity in Patients with Acute Major Depression. Neuroscience 169:415– 421.

Pause, B, Miranda, A, Goder, R. Aldenhoff, et al. (2001) Reduced Olfactory Performance in Patients with Major Depression. Journal of Psychiatric Research 35(5): 271-277.

Peacock, B, Scheidere, D, Kellermann, H. (2017) Biomolecular Aspects of Depression: A Retrospective Analysis. Comprehensive Psychiatry February 73:168–180.

Perera T, Park S, Nemirovskaya Y (2008) Cognitive Role of Neurogenesis in Depression and Antidepressant Treatment. Neuroscientist 14(4):326 –338.

Physical Activity Guidelines for Americans Midcourse Report Subcommittee of the President's Council on Fitness, Sports & Nutrition. (2012) *Physical Activity Guidelines for Americans Midcourse Report: Strategies to Increase Physical*

Activity Among Youth. Washington, DC: U.S. Department of Health and Human Services.

Sathyanarayana, R, Sha, M, Ramesh, B, Jagannatha, K (2008). Understanding Nutrition, Depression, and Mental illnesses. Indian Journal of Psychiatry. 50(2): 77-82.

Schwartz TL, Santarsieri D. (2016) Neural Implications of Psychotherapy, Pharmacotherapy, and Combined Treatment in Major Depressive Disorder. Mens Sana Monogr. Jan-Dec;14(1):30-45.

Shin, E, Seo, K, Lee, S, Jang, J, et al. (2016) Massage with or without Aromatherapy for Symptom Relief in People with Cancer. Cochrane Database Systematic Review. June (6):

Siqueria, C. (2016) Antidepressant Efficacy of Adjunctive Aerobic Activity and Associated Biomarkers in Major Depression: A 4-Week, Randomized, Single-Blind, Controlled Clinical Trial. PLoS One. 11(5): e0154195.

Strobel, L. (1998) *The Case for Christ: A Journalist's Personal Investigation of the Evidence for Jesus.* Grand Rapids:Zondervan.

U.S. Department of Health and Human Services and U.S. Department of Agriculture. (2015) 2015 – 2020 Dietary Guidelines for Americans. 8th Edition. December.

Zschucke, E. (2013) Exercise and Physical Activity in Mental Disorders: Clinical and Experimental Evidence. J Prev Med Public Health 46:S12-S21.

Movie Reference:

Atchison, D. (Director). (2006). *Akeelah and the Bee* [Film]. Santa Monica, CA: Lionsgate films.

Resource Section

Organizations

Mental Health America

MHA provides online educational resources, including screening tools and programs tailored to a variety of locations including schools and the work place.

500 Montgomery Street, Suite 820

Alexandria, VA 22314

Phone: 703-684-7722

Toll free: 800-969-6642

http://www.mentalhealthamerica.net/

Crisis Text Line – Text MHA 741741

National Alliance on Mental Illness

NAMI has programs that help pair individuals and family members with mental illness with others who have similar experiences. Family-to-Family and Peer-to-Peer programs are the popular and informative. They also host the NAMI Faithnet interfaith resource network.

3803 N. Fairfax Drive, Suite 100

Arlington, VA 22203

Phone: 703-524-7600

HelpLine: 800-950-6264

http://www.nami.org

Crisis Text Line – Text NAMI to 741-741

National Suicide Prevention Lifeline

Call 800-273-TALK (8255)

Naturopathic medicine
If considering a Naturopathic approach, check to see if your state offers licensed professionals, as well as their possible prescribing privileges:

Federation of Naturopathic Medicine Regulatory Authorities (FNMRA)
President: Anne Walsh, Oregon Board of Naturopathic Medicine
9220 SW Barbur Blvd., Ste 119, #321
Portland, OR 97219
Phone: 503-452-2953
www.fnmra.org
info@fnmra.org

Herbal Medicine
Other than in California, there are no state regulations regarding licensure. However, the American Herbalists Guild has an Herbalist Registry and the American Botanical Council serves as a research and educational organization.

American Herbalists Guild
P.O. Box 3076
Asheville, NC 28802-3076
Phone: 617-520-4372
Email: office@americanherbalistsguild.com
http://www.americanherbalistsguild.com/

American Botanical Council
6200 Manor Rd, Austin, TX 78723
Phone: 512-926-4900
Email: abc@herbalgram.org
http://abc.herbalgram.org

Donna Koczaja, MS
Herbalist
Phone: 240-353-8754
Email: greenhavenliving@gmail.com
http://www.greenhavenliving.com/

U.S. Food and Drug Administration

See website of Guidance and Regulation of Supplements and Herbal medicines where they also recommend following Good Manufacturing practice

10903 New Hampshire Avenue
Silver Spring, MD 20993
Phone: 1-888-INFO-FDA (1-888-463-6332)
http://www.fda.gov/Food/GuidanceRegulation/Guid anceDocumentsRegulatoryInformation/DietarySupp lements

Self-Care Resources

The University of Buffalo SUNY School of Social Work has a website with basic information on Self Care including assessments and ideas.

https://socialwork.buffalo.edu/resources/self-care-starter-kit.html

Written Materials

Mind Over Mood: Change How You Feel By Changing the Way You Think by Dennis Greenberger, Christine A. Padesky,

The Mind Over Mood workbook introduces the reader to the concept of Cognitive Behavior Therapy and includes worksheets such as Thought Logs to monitor thoughts, feelings and behaviors.

Battlefield of the Mind by Joyce Meyer

This book goes through principles to help deal with the thoughts that enter the mind and appropriately re-focus them.

Apps and Podcasts

NAMI Air is a "safe and anonymous app to air and share your experiences"

YouVersion Bible App contains a variety of subject-based content, some of which include links to audio or video presentations. You can search for content on for multiple areas of concern, including Depression.

Note from the Author

Dear Reader,

Thank you for allowing me to share this part of your journey with you. My purpose was to give you information that would help you see real change in your life. Hopefully, it was just the right amount of information for you. I would love to hear from you. Please let me know if you found value in the book and what other materials would be helpful. You may reach me at LedLifePublishing@gmail.com. I am excited for how far you have come and for journey ahead of you. I look forward to hearing how you far you have progressed and sharing further in your joys!

Be blessed,

Dr. Bergina

CPSIA information can be obtained
at www.ICGtesting.com
Printed in the USA
BVOW09s1324110318
510150BV00001B/87/P